# BEND

## DON'T
## BREAK

'I truly enjoyed this book – what a rollercoaster of emotions. Frank faces up to Parkinson's by calling on every challenge he has had on the running track and in life. If you can rise to a challenge in one area, then you have a greater chance of dealing with any others that come your way. He accepts adversity head-on, always finding a way forward. We all need a stabiliser in life and Frank has shown throughout his life that when the ship's about to keel over you need to take a deep breath and lean the other way.'

SONIA O'SULLIVAN, Olympic silver medallist,
Irish middle-distance runner

'His bravery, his fight to survive and the manner in which he's dealt with adversity is simply awe-inspiring.'

EAMONN COGHLAN, Three-time Olympian,
Irish middle-distance runner

'Frank's will and determination is parallel to our small, great nation, which continually punches above its weight. It takes an exceptional individual, coming from a tiny nation on the western periphery of Europe, to excel as a world-class middle-distance runner, as it's a brutal and hard-fought field. And if that wasn't a superhuman effort enough, Frank's resilience is tested once again when he is diagnosed with early onset Parkinson's disease at just forty-eight years of age. His truly remarkable and humbling account of his struggles with Parkinson's, and his undying will not to let it define him, make this a compelling read.'

SEÁN ÓG Ó hAILPÍN, Cork All-Ireland winning hurler and inter-
county footballer

'I found it almost impossible to put down, beautifully written.'
STEVE OVETT, Olympic gold medallist,
British middle-distance runner

*'Bend, Don't Break* is an inspirational book, the story of a man making the most of a life sentence. The hours I spent reading about [Frank's] experience were up there with the best use of my time [this year].'
DAVID WALSH, *The Sunday Times*

'I thoroughly recommend Frank's book. As a fellow Parkinson's sufferer, diagnosed in 1995, I learned a lot from Frank's journey and perspective. Compelling reading.'
JOHN WALKER, Olympic gold medallist,
New Zealand middle-distance runner

'I loved *Bend, Don't Break*. I appreciated Frank's resilience, unqualified courage and servant leadership. This book was both life changing and reaffirming.'
KEVIN WHITE, Former Athletic Director of Notre Dame and
Duke Universities

'Frank O'Mara's story is amazing, and he tells it with candour, humour and nuggets of wisdom we all can use.'
KATHY SULLIVAN, Scientist, astronaut, explorer

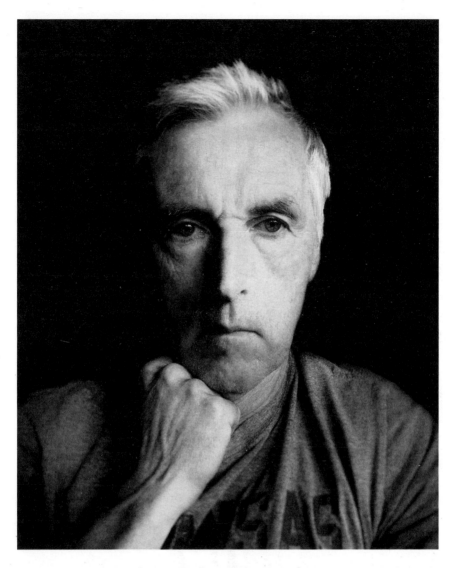

FRANK O'MARA is a former Irish runner. A three-time Olympian, he was twice World Indoor Champion in the 3,000 metres. Frank gained post-graduate degrees from the University of Arkansas and went on to have a successful career in the US wireless industry. He was diagnosed with early onset Parkinson's disease at the age of forty-eight.

# FRANK O'MARA

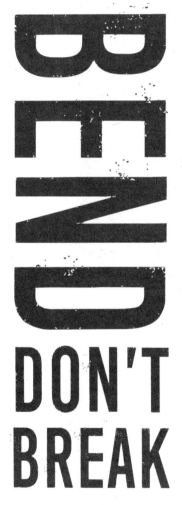

# BEND
# DON'T
# BREAK

## A MEMOIR OF ENDURANCE

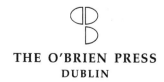

THE O'BRIEN PRESS
DUBLIN

First published in 2024 by
The O'Brien Press Ltd,
12 Terenure Road East, Rathgar, Dublin 6, D06 HD27 Ireland.
Tel: +353 1 4923333; Fax: +353 1 4922777
E-mail: books@obrien.ie
Website: obrien.ie

The O'Brien Press is a member of Publishing Ireland
ISBN: 978-1-78849-437-3
Text © copyright Frank O'Mara, 2024
The moral rights of the author have been asserted
Copyright for typesetting, layout, editing, design
© The O'Brien Press Ltd

8 7 6 5 4 3 2 1
28 27 26 25 24

Cover design and internal design by Emma Byrne
Picture credits:
Front cover photograph (and author photograph p 4) by Frank O'Mara; Back cover
photograph courtesy of ASICS.
P 19 'Ringing the Opening Bell on the NYSE', courtesy of NYSE ; P 63, 'CEO of AWCC'
courtesy of *Arkansas Democrat-Gazette*.; P 90 '1977 Irish Schools final', photograph by
Kieran Clancy. P 225 Used with permission of Mayo Foundation for Medical Education and
Research, all rights reserved. P 245 'Penn Relays' photograph by Dave Coskey; used with
permission. P 254, 'Hiking, Antarctic' photograph by Peter Wei; used with permission.
All other images author's own.
Every effort has been made to trace holders of copyright material used in this book,
but if any infringement has inadvertently occurred, the publishers ask the
copyright holders to contact them immediately.
A donation will be made to Parkinson's charities from the author's royalties.
Visit benddontbreak.live for more details

Printed and bound by CPI Group (UK) Ltd, Croydon, CR0 4YY
The paper in this book is produced using pulp from managed forests.

Published in
DUBLIN
UNESCO
City of Literature

Great Irish books
O'BRIEN
obrien.ie

## Dedication

I wish I had never met a single neurologist or neurosurgeon, but fourteen years into this saga, I have the contact details for many. This book is dedicated to all those from whom I have received treatment or counsel, but especially to Drs Lee Archer, Erika Petersen and Rohit Dhall at the University of Arkansas for Medical Sciences (UAMS) in Little Rock, Arkansas and Dr Kendall Lee at the Mayo Clinic in Rochester, Minnesota. Without your care many of us would not have the tools to cope.

# CONTENTS

# SOMETIMES YOU HAVE TO ACCEPT THE UNBELIEVABLE

The event that finally forced me to face reality didn't happen in a doctor's office or a hospital.

I didn't feel the true weight of my diagnosis until my friend Gary Taylor came over to check on us at home.

Gary was aware that I'd been struggling with some sort of malady for months. He'd followed my effort to treat my issue as a sports injury. When my sports medicine specialist said it might be a little more complicated than that, I saw a spine-doctor to rule out spinal stenosis. Next up, the neurologist.

Gary knew I'd seen a neurologist earlier that week, but he didn't know what, if anything, we'd learned.

The doctor had performed what seemed to be perfunctory tests, nothing elaborate: routine hand motions, finger tapping, foot stomping, and basic balance and gait tests. The exam only lasted about ten minutes. The doctor's response had been quick and precise. 'I've seen this often enough to recognise it. There is a slowness in your movement on the left side. I'm sorry to have to tell you this. You have Parkinson's disease.'

I took his assessment with a degree of scepticism.

'What baffles me is, I came in with a running problem and I'm leaving with an old person's neurological disease,' I said.

The doctor just shook his head, but I pressed on. 'I'm *only forty-eight years old.*'

The doctor had then proposed a way I might postpone reality a little longer. 'I suggest that you take a drug called Sinemet, which is used to treat the symptoms of the disease,' he said. 'If you see an improvement, then you know you have Parkinson's. If you don't, then you know I'm wrong.'

I didn't know Dr Archer very well at that point, but I appreciated that he refrained from adding, 'I think you'll find that I am right.' Since then, I have given him many opportunities to say, 'I told you so,' but he never has.

On my way home from the neurologist, I had called my wife, Patty, and rattled on about having no visible symptoms, so what improvement would I even look for? She humoured me, which only served as reinforcement in my confused mind. As I saw it, I was just trying to get to the bottom of a chronic injury that prevented me from running and was now beginning to interfere with my walking.

'I don't have a single symptom the doctor could point to,' I persisted. 'I don't even have a tremor!'

As usual, Patty gave wise counsel. 'Why don't I pick up the medicine this afternoon, and you can give it a go like he's suggested?' she said. 'Why don't you try it?'

It was a few days later that Gary came by. I was upstairs when I heard him knock on the front door. I looked out the window and saw his truck parked out front. I thought he'd come by to discuss the startup of a running store. I wasn't a great fan of retail, so I was a little anxious about the conversation. It took me a few minutes to finish what I was doing, then I headed down to the kitchen.

As I descended the stairs, I heard voices and what sounded like sobbing. I stopped for a moment to listen and heard Gary's voice above my wife's muffled crying. I listened a little while longer, but their hushed voices were indecipherable. I continued down to the landing and turned the corner into the kitchen. Neither Gary nor Patty had heard me coming and my sudden appearance surprised them.

I felt like I'd crashed the party. The look on both their faces said it all. I could tell they were guilty of some deceit. Gary had his arm around Patty. If I hadn't known them both so well, I would have thought they were about to admit to a clandestine affair. I almost excused myself for interrupting. Confused, uncertain what emotion to deploy, I just peered at them. I will never forget the stricken looks on their faces.

Gary saw my perplexed stare and broke the silence. 'God, I am *so sorry*, Frank!'

It was then I realised what they were trying to hide from me. Patty had told Gary about my doctor's visit earlier in the week.

'So, you heard the news, did you?' I blurted out.

'I did, and I feel awful for both of you,' Gary replied.

Then he hugged me. It was one of those long hugs, the kind given when no words are readily available. Gary clinched tighter before he released me.

'You're strong,' he said. 'You got this.'

I wanted to impress on him my disbelief, to tell him how wrong the doctor must have been, how little evidence there was to support the diagnosis. After all, Gary was a runner and should know about injuries. But there was a firmness in his eyes and a resolve in his voice that caused me to repress the urge.

There was nothing else to do except cry. We sobbed.

Their faces shocked me to my core. It was especially horrifying to see my beautiful wife look so worried. She had accepted my disbelief because she knew it might take time to accept, let alone digest the news. On the other hand, she had no reason to disbelieve the doctor. That was the moment I knew I was facing a monstrous challenge. I couldn't keep reality at bay any longer.

I had early onset Parkinson's disease at the age of *forty-eight*.

## CHAPTER I

# COME AND GET YOUR LOVE

**S**uch is the all-consuming nature of this odious disease that it tries to define your life. Today, I am first and foremost a Parkinson's warrior. My everyday schedule consists of one task above all others: do battle with the disease and slow its progression.

Before PD, I'd have described myself in the simplest terms as an athlete and a businessman, with a wonderful wife, three beloved sons – Jack, Colin and Harry – and friends all over the world.

After showing some mettle as a schoolboy runner in Limerick, Ireland, I earned a track and field scholarship to the University of Arkansas in 1978, part of a wave of Irish runners recruited by schools in the United States during the 1970s and 1980s. I took full advantage of the opportunity. My college track coach was a fellow Irishman, John McDonnell. John's teams won forty-two National Collegiate Athletic Association (NCAA) team titles, and he became the winningest coach in NCAA history. Back in 1979, he had yet to have a top-ten finish, but I can assure you that he was no less determined then than he was during the subsequent halcyon years. The expectation is that scholarship athletes perform at a superior level, but I took some time to hit my stride. I suffered from the oppressive heat when I arrived in Arkansas. That fall I ran straight into my first Indian summer.

Three weeks after our arrival in Fayetteville, fellow freshman Dave Taylor and I were especially struggling. It was boiling hot that afternoon and we were trailing home, a long way behind the others. We had been dripping wet, but strangely our skin began to dry up; we had learned over the last few weeks that dehydration meant trouble. By now we were walking, close to staggering, when suddenly we saw a sign for Malkowski Beverages. We were convinced it was a mirage, so we approached in disbelief. It turned out to be real. We could hear muffled voices and the hum of a forklift truck. There was activity – good. We stuck our heads through the open loading doors and were approached by a puzzled foreman. They found our accents difficult, and with slurry speech from dehydration, we were especially hard to follow. Fortunately, our body language said it all, and he rushed off to fetch us a cold drink.

Apparently, water could not be found; he returned instead with two cans of beer. We were in a beverage company alright, an alcoholic beverage company. What choice did we have? We happily drank the beer. It was liquid, and it was cold. Employees gathered around these two foreigners in nylon running shorts, shirts long ago discarded, allegedly speaking English. We must have been quite a sight. After a short rest and two empty cans, we began a slow, laborious slog back to campus. We may not have been inebriated, but we were close, and I have no doubt we appeared that way. Anyone who saw us in the last mile should have pulled over and checked on us. But runners were not a regular sight in Fayetteville in the seventies, let alone two semi-clad drunken runners.

Eventually, we appeared back in the locker room totally spent. Our teammates, showered and dressed, laughed and guffawed as we staggered straight into cold showers. We took our shoes off, but that was all.

I continued to struggle to establish momentum in my college athletics career for the first year, but I ultimately became the first University of Arkansas athlete to win an NCAA outdoor title during Coach McDonnell's era and second ever after Clyde Scott, who won the 110-metre hurdles way back in 1948. I don't know exactly why it was such a battle at first, other than that I was overworked the first few years and more than a little overwhelmed. But I kept plugging away and never lost my conviction.

My friends like to say I 'retired' from Arkansas in 1994, after eleven years in the classroom, with degrees in engineering, business and law. In my defence, I was a professional athlete; I had time on my hands.

Truth is, while I loved being an athlete and enjoyed a fair share of athletic success, I also faced an equal measure of disappointment. When I look back on my athletic career, I often think of the regrets, all the 'could haves' and 'would haves' that torment me. If I had only stayed closer to the leader at the Europeans in Stuttgart or if I had taken the lead from John Ngugi at the World Championships in Rome.

My fellow countrywoman and good friend, Sonia O'Sullivan, has asserted that it takes balance to be good, but you need to be unbalanced to be great. I think she means that your entire life must be devoted to sport. To be the best ever, you need a crazed application, a *'nothing else matters'* approach. I spent much of my athletic prime in the classroom. I didn't feel at the time I was hedging my bets, but in hindsight it likely demonstrates that I wasn't one hundred per cent committed. That would have required every waking hour to be dedicated to athletics. That wasn't the case with me; I had exams to take and papers to write. Sonia asserts that the imbalance in her life made her the force she became. She reached the pinnacle of achievement and stayed there for the best part of a decade. I worked really hard and sacrificed more than most, but I knew there was a ton of living after athletics was over. I guess I had balance.

In my case, that dream was racing around a track anti-clockwise for four laps as quickly as possible. I had some great results over my career. I ran a mile in 3:51.06 in 1986 and I won two World Championships. But any sense of achievement was tarnished by the failures, many caused by injury.

In a sport measured absolutely by time, mine began to run out. Like many high-level athletes, in the end it was injuries – and all the wear and tear on the body – that gave me no choice but to retire.

So, I turned toward a career in long pants.

Fortunately, I was prepared, not only with a master's in business administration (MBA) and a Juris Doctor (JD) degree in law, but also with an appetite for commercial enterprise. Business was in my DNA.

My father had been a serial entrepreneur who owned many small businesses. His last venture was a successful soft-drinks business, which he owned and operated in my hometown in the southwest of Ireland. I was brought up working holidays and weekends in the bottling plant. Initially, I fed the massive glass-bottle washing machine, a particularly arduous task. I graduated to driving the forklift, which I found easier than standing in front of the giant mouth of a washer as it ingested a dozen bottles at a time and disgorged steam at skin-sizzling temperatures. Eventually, I made sales calls in a pickup truck. On occasion, I made collections calls as well. I became well-versed in the vagaries of business.

In January of 1997, I joined Alltel, a wireline company founded in 1946 as Allied Telephone Company in Little Rock, Arkansas. My tenure began when the wireless industry was in its infancy. Over the next decade, Alltel became one of the largest wireless, or mobile network, carriers in the United

States, with nearly fourteen million customers and $10 billion in annual revenue. In two years, I was a corporate officer leading the human resources team. Eventually, I found myself in charge of the customer service, sales, and marketing teams.

The wireless mobile network industry in the 2000s turned out to be a great outlet for someone hoping to keep his competitive juices flowing. I was soon swept up in a dogfight as Alltel took on the emerging players in the field. We drove hard to acquire new customers, launch new devices, and lower our customer churn rate. Every day, there were deadlines and sales quotas to meet, network parameters to account for, new technologies to review and select. It was a constant battle, with our successes and failures publicly reported quarterly to the markets. A poor result would rile analysts and shareholders and could have devastating consequences for share prices, much more catastrophic than losing a race.

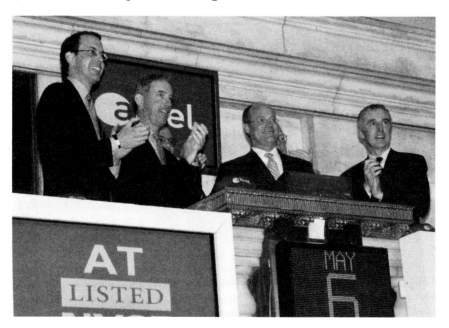

6 May 2006. Ringing the Opening Bell on the NYSE to celebrate Alltel's new logo.

I enjoyed seeing our team ranked against the other players in the field, much like rankings in sports. I especially loved that Alltel wasn't afraid to tussle with its bigger rivals, and that I wasn't, either. When I'm honest about my athletics career, there were a couple of times when I may have shied away from challenging the biggest dogs. Not so in my business career.

And then, at the height of our success in the wireless industry, my life – the life I'd wanted, for the most part, and the life I'd made for myself – suddenly came under attack.

I'd like to tell you that I immediately identified my new challenge and faced it head on. That's not what happened. Mine was a slow turning, a reluctant capitulation to reality.

My new life really began when I took that first dose of artificial dopamine, Sinemet. Even then, my Parkinson's journey remained full of disbelief and distrust as I grasped at alternate theories, looking for an escape hatch. At times, I shut off common sense, wilfully ignored conventional wisdom, and disregarded the competence of others. Against hard evidence, I refused to accept my burden, my ever-growing list of disabilities. I would bend, but not break.

It has taken me a while to find some peace.

But I have found peace. And acceptance. I've found hope, tasted success, felt joy. I have also come to recognise the many important lessons I'd already learned from my life's experiences before PD. What I had once seen as failures, especially my athletic disappointments, I have come to see in a very different light as a Parkinson's warrior. Beyond the track, my experiences as a son and sibling, husband and father, employer and employee, strengthen my resolve and sharpen my focus against Parkinson's daily. Skills developed before PD have become essential weapons in my current struggle.

Through Parkinson's, I learned to have gratitude for the person I was, as well as the person I am becoming. The disease is now a big part of my life's narrative, but it is not the only part. I came into this fight with the ability to focus on the process, to compartmentalise and not worry about the unknown, to never let despondency get a foothold.

The story of how I acquired those abilities and how I've applied them throughout my life is clearer to me now than ever before. And, in spite of Parkinson's, my story isn't finished yet.

The first indication that something nefarious had invaded my body appeared on 9 January 2009, the day after Verizon Wireless completed its purchase of Alltel Wireless, the largest mobile phone provider gobbling up the fifth largest. I should have taken heed of those early signs, but I was preoccupied with what I thought was a more imminent threat.

The team I worked with had done a tremendous job keeping Alltel relevant against the behemoths, AT&T and Verizon, whose advertising budgets were well over a billion dollars a year. We were a gritty underdog who wouldn't stop nipping at their heels. We poked fun at the big guys in award-winning creative. And everything was going swimmingly. The Alltel sponsored Number 12 Dodge had won NASCAR's biggest prize, the Daytona 500, the previous February. We had hosted Superbowl 39 at Alltel Stadium in Jacksonville, Florida. We were a national player in the industry.

Then, suddenly, the big guy took the ball, and the game was over. Our teams and our almost fourteen million customers were now part of Verizon Wireless. Mind you, it cost Verizon the princely sum of $28.1 billion.

I was the Chief Commercial Officer at Alltel, a job I relished. Unfortunately, Verizon already had more than one of me. I understood that the wireless giant preferred its own people. Still, I was disappointed with the treatment I received when my team and I visited the Verizon campus in New Jersey to brief the acquirers about operations. My onetime rivals could at least have feigned interest, but instead they displayed the touch of a blacksmith. After introductions and a brief overview of each department, we broke into smaller groups to discuss deal-related synergies. I was left with no peer, nobody to talk to. My counterparts just vanished.

So, I spent the day wandering around the venerable old campus, the former headquarters of AT&T.

Some months later in early January, the deal closed. A few of us were notified that our use-by date had expired, and we should pack up and exit. It was not easy strolling the floors that we once hurried on, saying goodbye to colleagues who had poured their heart and soul into the enterprise.

The day after I discovered time was up on my Alltel sojourn, I met a couple of friends, Mark Andersen and Gary Taylor, for a five-mile run on the river trail in Little Rock. The conversation was routine that morning. We chatted about the usual stuff: family and sport. Abruptly, Mark asked, 'What's going on with you this morning, Frank?'

Based on an assumption that he'd missed the Verizon news, my response was surly. 'You don't know about the Verizon deal closing? What rock have you been under?'

'Of course I know about that,' Mark replied, running a step or two behind me. 'Wasn't it in this morning's paper? I was wondering what's up with your leg?'

'My leg? There's nothing wrong with my leg.'

'It looks like your left leg is about to catch your right calf; the swing-through seems to be catching in the hip area.'

He motioned to Gary to slow down and get behind me.

'Gary, get back here and check this out.'

He obliged. I humoured them, still more distracted by the ramifications of the Verizon acquisition than concerned about a critique of what had been, after all, a serviceable running stride. They concurred that something was amiss, but said so gingerly. One didn't need a PhD in psychology to determine I was irritable that morning.

A mile later, PD struck its first memorable blow. As my left leg moved forward, my left foot clashed with my right calf and almost brought me crashing down. It happened a couple of more times in quick succession. One of my companions, looking for a reprieve from a not exactly torrid pace, suggested that we stop and stretch. It seemed a realistic accommodation.

Although I was in my own little world, focused mostly on my uncooperative leg, I remember watching my friends' warm breath being expelled into the crisp, frosty air. A minute later, the body heat from their shoulders and upper backs created the same effect. It was a gorgeous Saturday morning, typical of January in Arkansas, when cold weather from the north challenges warm weather from the gulf. A sharp bite of chilly weather battled a full sun, the sun doomed to suffer defeat. We returned to the run before conditions worsened.

My companions weren't thrilled when my malady returned less than half a mile later. I requested another time out. They had to endure two further stops in the last kilometre. It reminded me of NASCAR, when a race car is forced to make a stop in the closing laps for a splash of gas.

'That looks like a problem that you need to address,' Mark said, when we arrived back at the parking lot.

'It's probably nothing,' I responded.

We were all beginning to shiver as we stood there, barely sheltered from the icy wind by a minivan. I was in no frame of mind to indulge anyone's proclivity for worry. With only the intention of ending the conversation so we could get in our cars and crank up the seat warmers, I added, 'I'll go see a physical therapist on Monday.'

As I drove off, I noticed that Gary and Mark were huddled together. Gary was sitting against the driver's seat with the door open and his feet on the ground. He was giving Mark a proper listening to. Mark appeared animated, and there was no doubt he was doing the talking. Many years later, Gary told me that Mark had raised the spectre of a neurological cause to my just-revealed injury.

Mark is an MD whose advice I am inclined to heed; but on the topic of overuse injuries, I considered myself an expert. When I was competing, it seemed like I was recovering from or working around an injury most of the time – it's part of a runner's life. So, this issue just seemed like more of the same. I regarded it more as an inconvenience than a true injury. I saw a massage therapist every week. The problem persisted, introducing itself earlier and earlier in runs as time passed by. One day in early spring, it showed up when Patty and I were out walking not far from our home in Little Rock.

There was a clear sky that morning, a clear sky that might last another week or so, before the earth and every living thing would be covered in a grimy layer of yellow, menacing pollen. There were times when you could see clouds of it billowing through the air. Anything that is stationary for even a moment will be doused in this sneeze-inducing stuff, rendering outside activity next to impossible for the majority of April. The cleanup from this mess must cost households millions across the South. It certainly keeps the car washes busy.

Patty could have been a professional walker. She sets an enviable pace, one that requires a degree of effort. It's exercise to her, not leisure. If you're not careful, she'll gain a step on you ... and then a step becomes two. About halfway through our walk, I fell two steps behind her ... and then three. That's when it struck: the identical sensation I had experienced in my runs. My left leg refused to play its role, to operate within the plane of motion required. As a result, my left foot hit my right calf when that leg was pulling through and my right leg was planted.

I stopped and called to Patty, 'Give me a moment to see if I can stretch this problem out.' Patty slowed to a stop and waited.

'Do you think this is the same issue you have running?' she asked.

This was worrisome. The problem had progressed in my running and was now manifest in my walking.

'Maybe it's a fluke,' I replied. 'If it returns after this stretch, we'll know it's not a fluke.'

Patty will have been my wife for thirty-three years come October. She says our anniversary is October 6 or 7. I can't remember. I consider the exact date to be irrelevant: we chose the first Saturday in October as our wedding day, so we should observe the first Saturday as *the* day. It's far easier to remember and celebrate. Thankfully, we can disagree without irritating one another.

I first saw Patty in church, while we were both undergraduates at the University of Arkansas. Jokingly, a friend had volunteered me to be an altar boy. It was sheer providence that Patty was in church that day and saw me on the altar. Although I had no idea who she was or how to meet her, I remained keenly interested from afar. Then, with approximately a week of

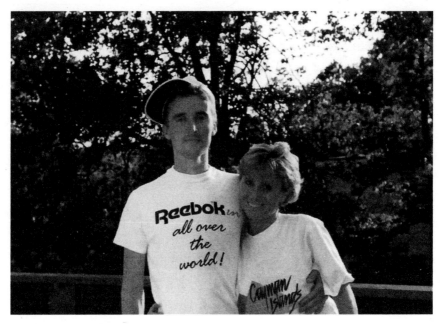

16 October 1985. With Patty Olberts shortly after we began dating.

school remaining, I spotted her walking into a sorority house on campus. I immediately called a classmate, Molly Inhofe, who was a member of that sorority and asked if she knew the mystery girl. Not only did Molly know her, they were roommates.

With an introduction from Molly, I asked Patty out that weekend. She demurred; said she was all booked. The only time she could fit me in was Thursday … for lunch. There'd be no primetime airing for me.

I thought we had a great time at lunch, convinced that I'd met the woman I would marry. Patty didn't leap to the same conclusion. That evening, I went to a Razorback baseball game, only to see my future wife out on a date. She caught my eye for a second and immediately turned away without even a hint of a smile.

But I was not discouraged. I wrote to her numerous times from various countries that summer. I even sent her a postcard from Iceland in a vain attempt to woo her. She was impressed enough to respond, *once*. Still, I wasn't discouraged.

The next fall, Patty, Molly, and I were all in business school together. Finally, with Molly's endorsement, I charmed Patty into dating me. I know she has loved me unconditionally since, albeit with me fifth in line after our three sons and our Goldendoodle.

I would need several volumes more to enumerate all the things I love about Patty, but here are an important few: I love how pragmatic she is, and how devoted she is to family. She is amazingly even-keeled and seems not to suffer mood swings. She doesn't play games or keep score.

Once, when my Alltel team and I were choosing an advertising agency, one of the competing agencies submitted an idea centred on the theme of love. It went something like, 'We so love our customers that we provide them (insert a relevant value proposition) and in return our customers love us.' The agency suggested we license the seventies hit song by Redbone called 'Come and Get Your Love.' Of all the ideas the agencies pitched, this was the one favoured by the marketing team. I was sceptical, however. I felt that the term 'love' was overused, particularly in the United States. I noted, for example, that people use 'love you' as a salutation at the end of phone calls, rendering the words, in most contexts, almost meaningless.

When several of us met to choose the winning agency, someone challenged me to call my wife and end the call with, 'Love you.' I was up for the challenge. I needed to rid myself of doubt about the favoured campaign, get over my reticence. So, I hit #1 on speed dial and within three rings, Patty picked up. I made some small talk, tried to sound casual, but the other people in the room could tell I was labouring. I had to talk long enough to make 'Love you' sound like a throwaway comment. I made up something innocuous about a scheduling issue, then said, 'I have to run.'

'Alright. See you tonight then,' Patty responded.

After a long, awkward pause, I tried to recover, adding, 'hmmm, well, there's one more thing I want to tell you …'

'Go on then.'

'Love you,' I suddenly blurted out.

'*Is there something wrong with you?*' Patty replied, sounding more annoyed than perplexed.

'No, nothing wrong, I was just thinking … I'll just tell you tonight.'

'Alright, see you tonight.'

'Bye.'

I looked around the room. 'That went about how I expected,' I said, as my colleagues shook their heads. My teammates still favoured the Redbone idea, and I was wise enough to discount my own perspective. We chose the Love campaign, which turned out to be wildly successful.

Maybe Patty and I weren't the proper test sample to gauge the efficacy of an ad campaign, but we have always been a team. We are united, without conflict or agenda. We don't take each other's affection for granted. I love Patty more today than when I first met her, cherishing every moment we have spent together.

Given our understanding, when Patty witnessed my problem walking that early spring day, her concern began to heighten my own sense of alarm. Patty is also an exercise fiend, always has been. I knew that she understood the nature of injuries and the attendant frustrations of trying to play through them. The problem flared up at least twice more on that walk. Each time, Patty expressed her concern.

As you might have guessed, over the course of the coming months, my walking deteriorated in a similar gradual manner to my loss of running function. The more trouble I had, the more Patty urged me to see a doctor. Specifically, she suggested that I see a spine specialist.

Through sheer bull headedness and lots of delusion, I ignored all advice and continued to treat the issue as a soft tissue injury. Meanwhile, I lived on the hope that, when I got home to Ireland that summer, the Irish athletics medical staff would finally sort this thing out, just as they'd always done.

## CHAPTER 2

# PLAY THE ROLE AS SCRIPTED

**W**e arrived in Ireland in late June. I made a beeline for my friend Gerard Hartmann's home.

Gerard is a therapist of some renown, having participated as a member of the Irish and British medical staffs at six Olympic Games. In addition to amazingly powerful hands and a propensity for digging into muscle tissue to such a degree that I always wished I'd had a wooden spoon to bite down on, he also has an uncanny sixth sense.

In my running career, Gerard rescued my season on numerous occasions. When the time came, his opinion deeply influenced my decision to retire. Despite having achieved the qualifying time for the 1996 Olympic Games in Atlanta, I suffered from chronic leg pain on the left side caused by disc degeneration. By then I had run more than fifty thousand miles and the constant compression had worn out the lumbar vertebrae. When Gerard saw my MRI and discussed my skeletal system with orthopaedic doctors at the University of Florida, he gave it to me straight, recommending retirement.

Gerard and I have known each other since we were rivals in underage athletics in Ireland, then college students together at the University of Arkansas. We have both suffered through many injuries; together, we've tried all sorts of crazy schemes to get better, no matter how harebrained.

The maddest treatment Ger and I ever embraced was under the hands of a German therapist living on a lake in County Galway. We were home on Christmas break, both of us with knee injuries – the overuse kind that, no matter what you do, seem to take six to eight weeks to remedy. You could probably do nothing and get the same results, but you feel better about yourself if you're doing something – even if it only resembles therapy.

Ger discovered the German first, made the trip to Galway and reported when he got back.

'I went to Galway to see this therapist on Friday,' his pitch began.

'Well, what did you make of him?'

'You'll have to keep an open mind, but he may be onto something.'

'Why? What does he do that's so interesting?'

I should have read between the lines, but you cling to hope that the oddest treatment can be super effective.

'It's a bit strange. He does underwater massage, and he uses the tip of a *drumstick*,' Ger said. He sounded tentative.

'Is it worth my while driving up there? Have you seen any improvement?'

'You definitely should give him a shot.' Before I could respond, he added, 'I booked you an hour after my session on Monday.'

Monday arrived and Ger picked me up in his father's car. He had been cross-training that morning, as had I: he in the pool; me risking the country roads on a bicycle. Ger replayed the goings-on from the previous Friday visit to the German as we drove.

As I listened, any seed of doubt should have germinated; instead, wildflowers of hope bloomed: this could be just crazy enough to work!

We pulled into a drive, the gravel crunching under our tyres. There were a few dogs at the German's, and each inspired fear – particularly one who had been asleep under an upturned sailboat in the yard. We rolled to a stop. Only then could we appreciate the panic-inducing quality of their barks. Fortunately, the dogs' exultations alerted the German, who came to the side door and motioned us to come on in. He had that look that all owners of vicious dogs have, one that says, 'my dog is friendly', never mind the scary snarling.

I rolled down the window and asked, 'Can you put the dogs up, please?'

He said something in broken English with a thick-as-treacle German accent. I grasped the final statement: '*Alles GUT.*'

I turned to Ger. Before I could complain, he said, 'They will jump on you, but you'll be fine.'

'Easy for you to say. You have German shepherds at home.' Finally, the doctor's wife appeared and coaxed the excited creatures into the house. What a relief!

The doctor was friendly, eager to be of assistance. He quickly divined that I had patellar tendonitis – sometimes known as 'jumper's knee', this is an overuse injury resulting in inflammation of the tendon that connects the knee to the shin. Pretty standard to this point; then it took a turn toward strangeness. He asked me to sit on the treatment table, reached into a drawer and extracted a polished, wooden drumstick from a wide selection. He inspected the tip. He discarded his first selection and instead chose a stick with a broader tip and smiled ruefully. The German directed me to sit back on the table with my leg extended and he slowly applied the end of the drum to the lower quad muscles, especially the V-shaped muscle, *vastus intermedius*, between the *vastus lateralis* and *vastus medialis*. He went after it hard, pushing the unforgiving, sharp end of the drumstick deep into the tissue.

This modality was either revolutionary or highly foolish. But when you have been injured as often as I have been, desperation can take hold. When you watch your peers compete in your absence, you are prepared to endure a certain degree of pain to get back to competition.

Turns out, the German had more madness in store for me. He asked me to enter his hydro treatment room. This steamy room, with windows clouded in perspiration, was the centrepiece of the treatment protocol. Amid the dense fog hanging over the room, a large, raised hot tub held water that would hardly qualify as lukewarm. It was downright cool. The German instructed me to climb in the tub, then produced what looked like a firehose – a two-inch thick, not-your-garden-variety type hose – and attached it to a huge tap, the likes of which I'd never seen. Then he placed the hose in the tub, while adjusting the volume on the massive tap.

Suddenly, he applied the powerful stream of water to my quad. The fierce pressure from the hose pinned my leg to the bottom of the tub. He adjusted the impact by moving the mouth of the hose further away from my skin, all the time using a massage-type motion. I constantly had to brace myself or I would tumble around like clothes in a dryer. The pressure left my skin with an irritated sensation.

This was invasive treatment, I thought: just unusual enough that it may work. So, when the German suggested I make another appointment, I gladly acquiesced. Both Gerard and I returned on a couple of occasions but, sadly, saw little improvement. The episode illustrates how desperate we runners get as the weeks of injury and not training spin by.

Now, years past my athletic prime and facing new physical challenges, I took great comfort knowing I was in the hands of someone who understood the tribulations of injury and the paucity of treatment options. Gerard gave me quite a going-over that morning. When he completed the evaluation, he instructed me to get dressed and said he would be right back. In a short time, he returned, carrying two cups of tea. We sat down at a small table in his therapy room. Small, but tidy. Gerard is fastidious about organisation. He then offered the following, 'I see nothing wrong with your soft tissue. Plenty of flaccidity.'

'What about a hip impingement or spinal issues? Remember, I had that L4 and L5 issue when I ran,' I replied.

It was Gerard, after all, who had diagnosed the disc issue in my lower spine that led ultimately to my retirement from athletics. But here, he saw no connection.

'In my opinion there is nothing wrong with your skeletal or muscular systems. It's probably neurological. I'll send you to a sports specialist at the Santry Sports Surgery Clinic.'

This was the first mention of a neurological possibility.

Two weeks later, I found myself walking around Ireland's capital in a haze, dejected, with the sports doctor's concise verdict playing over and over in my mind, 'You have a serious issue in the basal ganglia area.'

The doctor had focused primarily on my balance. He instructed me to perform one-legged sitting squats, with my back against a wall. As I slid up and down the wall, my weight-bearing leg began to quiver. The quivering gradually spread to my unloaded leg, then to my arms. Before long, my body was shaking as if I were on an Irish beach in summer. The doctor made no comment, but ordered an MRI and sent me to the imaging department. After reviewing the images, he made his declaration: something neurological, involving the basal ganglia family.

When the words came out of the doctor's mouth, they initially didn't mean much to me. At that stage of my life, I was still unfamiliar with the geography of the brain, so I asked, 'What kind of conditions are associated with the *basal* ... whatever you called it?'

His response described a range of scary possibilities: 'It could be anything from Tourette's Syndrome to ALS – motor neurone disease.'

Anchored at one end by certain death, and at the other end of the range of possibilities – a lifetime of embarrassing tics and inappropriate comments – seemed like a walk in the park. And of course, there were the wide-open plains in between ...

The doctor couldn't be more precise. Although he was one of the most highly respected exercise and sports medicine physicians in the world, he was not a neurologist. I had hedged my bets a little, purposely choosing a sports doctor in a foolhardy effort to either delay a bad diagnosis or, more incredibly, influence the diagnosis itself. So badly had I wanted to avoid anything more serious than simple tendonitis.

I never saw that doctor again, save a few glimpses of him on television, treating members of the Irish rugby team. It's odd how strangers can play such pivotal roles in our lives.

I left his office bewildered. My train back to Limerick departed at 5:40, but instead of heading in the direction of Heuston Station, I wandered around Dublin aimlessly. I was alone and I was afraid. Truth is, no matter who cares about you, a battle for your health is very personal, and often lonely. To be sure, you would be absolutely lost without people who love you, many of whom would willingly swap places, but the struggle is ultimately yours and yours alone.

So, I meandered around the Fair City until I found myself sitting on the edge of the grass track in Trinity College, ruminating in the tranquil environment. As noisy as the city was, within the confines of the stone walls it felt like a sanctuary. Founded in 1592, Trinity is located right in the busiest section of the city centre. Once you pass through the massive original wooden doors – doors so huge, in fact, that a smaller door-within-the-door was added for pedestrian access – you enter an idyllic and inspirational world, embraced by the serenity of its carved stone edifices and beautiful cobbled paths.

At that moment, I began to shift my perspective, remembering that I must live in the present. I thought about my friend and fellow athlete Noel Carroll who worked out on the grass track within these confines during the summer months. He died much too early at fifty-six years old. I promised myself that I would play only the part currently assigned me. I might have a more difficult role later, but why get ahead of the script? At that moment, no one had decreed that I was in the grip of an awful disease, so why act like it? There would be ample opportunity to stress or worry if the situation merited it. I would not get ahead of myself. As I thought of Noel and his lost opportunities, of the loss his family must have felt, I vowed not to let the vision of a grim future interfere with my present-day plans.

I picked up my backpack and headed toward Heuston Station for the 7:50 train.

As I have come to realise, particularly in recent years, my kind of coping is heavily reliant on compartmentalisation. Every hour in every day is accounted for; every task and emotion have their place. There's a time for fun and a time for work; there's a place for joy and a place for worry.

This predilection for compartmentalisation, as well as my preference for order and capacity for self-discipline, revealed themselves when I was in secondary school. Where better to learn such coping skills than in a boarding school for boys? There, the peaceful coexistence of so many testosterone-rich teenagers required excessive degrees of discipline. How else would you keep order?

I had the great misfortune of going to boarding school at eleven years of age, an experience involving more than a few memorably fun moments, but ultimately marked by profound loneliness and feelings of separation. In boarding school, I learned that I could be surrounded by lots of people and still feel alone, that I could have lots of friends and still feel like a stranger. Boarding school can be a friendly environment, but not a loving one. That's because it is an institution that relies on rules and discipline to maintain control; it's not a home.

I remember my first night in the dormitory like it was yesterday. The school, St Munchin's College, was founded in 1776. The campus had recently moved from the city centre location to an idyllic spot overlooking the broad Shannon River. It was modern and up to date on the outside, but very spartan inside, almost industrial. To this eleven-year-old, it felt like an institution, certainly not my home. High ceilings, patterned concrete floors and an endless maze of corridors gave the school the feel of a government installation. The corridors were adorned with a huge array of team pictures, highlighting the school's emphasis on sports and its sterling reputation for success. At that moment, the school's past glories were of little consequence to me, as I tried to come to terms with this place being my abode for the next six years.

Upon our arrival at St Munchin's that afternoon, my mother and father had helped me prepare my 'cubicle.' A cubicle in the first-year dorm was scarcely six feet long and five feet wide, equipped with a small closet and a curtain we could pull across to create the barest impression of privacy. The curtain, made of dense, heavy fabric, emitted a high, piercing sound when dragged along its track. We were allowed to draw the blind only when getting dressed or undressed. The rest of the time, we were to remain in open view.

As my parents helped me unpack, I felt on edge. My mother tried to focus my attention on all the little motherly touches she'd added to the occasion. She'd sewn identification badges on all my clothing, the property of Francis A. O'Mara, had adorned my laundry bag with the handsewn word 'laundry', in case I forgot its purpose. She'd been particularly excited about a scratchy wool dressing gown she'd bought me. Repeatedly, I assured her I had no intention of ever wearing it.

My parents' solicitous behaviour seemed odd.

'Do you like your bed cover?'

I realised they were as anxious as I was.

'Oh yes, I love it!' I said, playing along.

'Your sisters picked it out,' my mother said, hoping a reference to my siblings *at home* might ease the tension.

I wanted to say something nice, but my nerves only produced sarcasm instead. 'Perhaps they'd like to take it to boarding school someday?'

Parents were to leave by 4:30; my anxiety multiplied as the appointed time grew closer. I don't remember much about our goodbyes, only the feeling of being left on my own. In utter disbelief, I watched them drive off, down the long, tree-lined driveway, across the cattle guard, and through the silver-painted gates bearing St Munchin's two-hundred-year-old crest: *Veritas in Caritate*, Truth in Charity. I was stunned when they didn't turn around, didn't come back saying the whole ordeal had been a prank. I stood there long after they disappeared from sight.

Somehow, I got through the next few hours. I remember receiving lots of instruction, lots of rules. After night prayers in the chapel, we went back to our dormitories.

Each dormitory had an assigned prefect, an upperclassman, who lived in a luxurious doublewide cubicle. He was a proxy for the Dean of Students, who held the ultimate power. The prefect was an enforcer. His nightly task of getting his charges to bed began with the ringing of a bell, indicating 'lights out' in five minutes. Five minutes later, as a second bell rang, the prefect would turn off the lights and patrol for any miscreants.

On my first night in the dormitory, the atmosphere reminded me of an aftermath of one of the bombings I'd grown up seeing reported on TV: people wandering around, shellshocked. Many of my peers lay in their beds, crying; a few had the audacity to torment those who were most distraught. One poor boy lay in his bed, sobbing, while his cubicle neighbour dangled some ticklish object in his face. The prefect clearly needed support. Suddenly, the dean, a formidable priest, arrived, rapidly and repeatedly turning the lights on and off until order was restored. Then the dean would walk around the dormitory slowly, inspecting each cubicle. He shone a torch on each bed to verify the occupant was appropriately bundled up and not in a pal's cubicle. Frequently, there were one or two missing and there had to be consequences for this transgression. Otherwise, the lunatics would run the asylum. A leather strap was the go-to weapon of choice.

That night, I had my first encounter with an affliction that I've dealt with ever since: insomnia.

When first deposited at St Munchin's, I felt abandoned. Later, I felt angry. Over time, I adapted to life away at school. There were some outrageous pranks worthy of documenting. There were great sporting moments worth recalling. But conversely, there were long dark nights in the study hall punctuated by night prayer in a cold chapel. I survived. In fact, I thrived sufficiently to become Second Prefect and make my mark as an athlete. But I can honestly say I was never happy. In many ways, boarding school was one long survival exercise.

Six years later, when I drove through those silver-painted gates for the last time, I was well versed in compartmentalisation. I'd developed the art of processing circumstances and dealing with accompanying emotions. I'd learned to assign various challenges and irritations to specific timeslots, when I'd deal with them appropriately, with clear focus and discipline.

Little did I know then how much I would come to need those skills.

I have long marvelled at the achievements of the explorer Ernest Shackleton, particularly the leadership he demonstrated throughout his famed saga in the Antarctic. Aboard the *Endurance*, he and his men were trapped in the ice through two blindingly dark winters. Understanding that idle minds are the devil's workshop, Shackleton ordered his crew to perform simple daily tasks, some of them purely made-up work. The sailors rearranged equipment and furniture, only to put it back in its original configuration the following week. Shackleton kept people busy. When he left Elephant Island in a desperate attempt to rescue his men, he instructed Frank Wild, who remained behind with twenty-one others, to have them assemble their meagre belongings every morning, as if, that day, they would be rescued. They did so every morning for four months until Shackleton returned. I would like to believe that Shackleton learned the nuances of discipline and compartmentalisation when he attended a boarding school, Dulwich College, in South England, albeit as a day pupil.

I became aware of Shackleton, who was born in Kildare, through my interest in another Irishman, Tom Crean, who hails from the same part of Ireland as my mother. Crean was on that fateful journey to the South Pole, accompanying Shackleton in a last-gasp dash to the whaling station on South Georgia Island for aid. To give credit where it is due, there was a third Irishman on the crazed final push to safety in that battered boat, Tim McCarthy from Kinsale. Three Irishmen in one of the epic survival stories of the century! Crean made numerous trips to the polar region and retired to county Kerry, where he owned a pub called The South Pole.

There is a rich history of polar adventure in Ireland, particularly in counties Kerry and Cork. For many years, these counties produced sailors for the Royal Navy, and some showed sufficient mettle to be chosen for harrowing trips to both poles. Patsy Keohane from Courtmacsherry was on the expedition team with Scott when he was beaten to the South Pole by Amundsen in 1911, as was Crean. Neither were chosen for the final push to the pole; that honour was only given to Royal Navy officers. Scott and team made it to the pole, but sadly they all perished on the return trip. Keohane was in the rescue party that found Scott's body.

That pub in the tiny village of Annascaul fuelled my fascination with the polar regions. My father took me there when I was a kid. We sat in a corner booth, and I sipped a Club Orange through a straw while my father had his brandy and ginger ale. My father was more interested in the *Irish Press* newspaper, so I was left to roam freely. The small pub was no longer owned by Crean by then, but it still bore his imprint. It was dark inside, difficult to see the polar memorabilia displayed in battered wooden cabinets. Bolts of light from the narrow windows occasionally pierced the darkness, illuminating tiny particles of dust floating in the air above dimpled concrete floors, randomly spotlighting parts of the collection – an ancient crampon here, a crinkled black and white photograph there.

I have visited that wonderful establishment on a number of occasions since I was a boy, inculcating a passion in me for the polar regions, igniting a dream to journey to the Antarctic, where I might see for myself the forlorn continent and understand the discipline necessary to survive on the ice through two winters. Unfortunately, due to the demands of my athletics and business careers, I'd never found time for such an expedition.

As Patty, the boys and I headed home to Arkansas from Ireland, I tried not to dwell on the growing likelihood that my future might well be determined by a significant, potentially deadly neurological disease. When my mind landed on one of my favourite subjects, however, I found neither distraction nor relief. Instead, I felt suddenly hopeless.

*I'll likely never make it to the South Pole,* I thought. *I'll never see Elephant Island.*

Compartmentalisation teaches a person to concentrate on the process and not fear the outcome.

When faced with a seemingly insurmountable task, you break it down into incremental steps. You learn never to allow the possible success or failure of an endeavour to influence your commitment to it. Neither success nor failure are within your control. You do, however, control your effort, method, application, decision-making, rigour, and level of thoughtfulness. These are learnable, repeatable skills that you can apply to any challenge. Sure, success is something to savour, something that can instil a certain kind of confidence. But it's not a skill or process you can use in any situation. Success without good underlying skill or process is no indicator of continued success. Failure, on the other hand, can at least motivate you to work harder to develop the right skill or process for use the next time you need to fight the good fight.

The Irish may be predisposed to compartmentalisation. In the movie classic *Gone with the Wind*, based on the 1936 novel by Margaret Mitchell, Scarlett O'Hara is initially distraught when Rhett Butler tells her he 'doesn't give a damn' about her. Scarlett's Irish temperament reveals itself when, after a few tears, she resolves to 'worry about that tomorrow.' The novel ends similarly: 'Tomorrow, I'll think of some way to get him back. After all, tomorrow is another day.' It's a classic Irish response. Further evidence of this cultural predisposition can be found in the Irish language. Instead of saying, 'I am happy,' we say, '*tá áthas orm*', or 'happiness is upon me', demonstrating that we don't expect the state of happiness to last. '*Tá brón orm*', or 'sadness is upon me', likewise implies that sadness also will pass. There is a time for everything: a time for worry and a time for hope. All these bouts of conflicting emotions may explain why the Irish are often considered a moody lot.

At the mere impulse to jump ahead and rule out any future voyage to Antarctica, I reflexively pushed away my fears. *Maybe I won't live long enough to see Elephant Island*, I thought as I looked out the plane window, *but I'll worry about that tomorrow.*

## CHAPTER 3

# DON'T FIXATE ON WORST-CASE SCENARIOS

B ack in the United States, I felt prepared to deal with whatever ailed me. In its assigned compartment, my health complaint – what I continued to regard as an elusive sports injury, despite the Dublin sports doctors' assessment – would receive my full and unflinching attention.

Whatever benefit my available coping skills provided me at the time, however, the prospect of a bad prognosis frightened the hell out of me.

Mark Andersen, the friend who'd first called attention to my uncoordinated stride, referred me to another former Arkansas track athlete, Dr Lee Archer, now the head of neurology at University of Arkansas for Medical Sciences. I knew of Lee as an athlete, but had no clue how successful Dr Archer had become in the medical world. Welcoming, disarmingly friendly, he has become my great ally and supporter over the years, his matter-of-fact manner somehow making what is difficult and scary seem manageable.

When we first met, I hardly regarded Dr Archer as a trusted ally. Rather, I so badly wanted to hear good news that I did everything I could to influence him, to throw him off the scent. After presenting tailored evidence to support my preferred diagnosis, I tediously explained that my only complaint was a running injury, which prevented me from controlling my left leg.

I purposely withheld the Irish doctor's opinion about my basal ganglia.

Dr Archer listened, then brushed away my defences with a nonchalant smile.

'Let's try a few easy tests,' he said.

'Okay, happy to!' My attitude was, *I'll ace your damn tests.*

'Let's begin with making fists. Hold out your right hand.' I held out my right hand and made a fist as directed.

'Now open your hand as wide as you can. Now clench and unclench as fast as you can.'

I followed his instructions exactly. With each movement, I felt my confidence grow.

'Now the other hand.' *Perfect*, I thought.

'Open your hands and hold your palms upward. Now turn your hand over so that the palm faces the floor.'

Easy as you please.

'Now, roll them over as quickly as you can.' *Nailed it.*

'Now the other hand, please.'

We did some additional tests on my feet, tapping the ground, pointing and flexing my toes. Dr Archer then instructed me to walk across the examination room, turn around, and walk back.

I didn't notice anything unusual with my gait, but I did notice that Dr Archer paid particular attention when I turned around.

The drill concluded with a series of challenges testing my balance. Again, in my opinion, there was nothing there to see.

'Sit down, Frank,' Dr Archer said.

The professional look on his face, as he pulled his chair closer and cleared his throat, should have telegraphed the gravity of the moment, but I was oblivious. In the long pause before Dr Archer began to speak, I *knew* I'd passed his tests.

'Frank, I'm sorry to have to tell you this. You have Early Onset Parkinson's disease (EOPD).'

'You can't be serious,' I said, my tone dismissive, almost arrogant.

'I am afraid I am,' Dr Archer continued. 'You have Parkinson's.'

'How can you tell?'

'I could tell when you walked in the room. The way you carried your arms gave it away.'

'You're serious? Really?' I couldn't reconcile his observations with my own physical experience, my own network of sensations and biofeedback, honed over decades spent training at the top level.

'The way you turned around was another giveaway. You took more steps than typical. Rather than pivoting, you kind of shuffled.'

'Let me try again. I'll do better this time,' I pleaded. This was my first meeting with Dr Archer, and I didn't yet know the depth of his experience and knowledge. I challenged him. 'Are you *sure*? How can you be *sure*?'

Dr Archer again reported what he'd seen. When I'd first walked into the room, he said, my arms weren't swinging naturally. He said there was rigidity in my carriage.

The tests turned out to be part of the Unified Parkinson's Disease Rating Scale (UPDRS), a scoring system used by clinicians and their patients to objectively track the disease's linear progression. Parkinson's is a degenerative disorder of the central nervous system, impairing motor function initially. As the disease progresses, that impairment becomes increasingly debilitating. Dr Archer explained the scale on the movement tests we'd done: the best score on each individual test is 0, or no signs of impairment; any positive score indicates some degree of impairment. Conversely, the worst score is 4.

'You scored ones in a number of categories,' Dr Archer said.

'Is there any other possible explanation? Could you be wrong?'

'It's possible,' he said, 'but I've seen this presentation before, and it's my opinion that you have PD. Now, I can refer you to an expert for a second opinion, but meanwhile here's what I suggest you do.'

He advised me to take a medicine that combats the symptoms of Parkinson's to see if I noticed any change.

I gave him a puzzled look and demanded, 'What symptom should I expect to see improvement in?'

'You should see an improvement in your walking problem,' he said, his tone still gentle.

The medicine Dr Archer suggested I take is an amino acid called L-dopa, a precursor to neurotransmitters dopamine, noradrenaline, and adrenaline, which the brain neglects to produce in sufficient quantities in Parkinson's sufferers. In high doses, L-dopa, or levodopa, causes nausea and vomiting. As a result, levodopa is usually given in combination with carbidopa, which enhances the levodopa and reduces the required therapeutic dose, preventing nausea and vomiting. The name brand of the medicine Dr Archer recommended was Sinemet, from the Latin word *sine* (without) and *ématos*, the Ancient Greek word for vomiting. As I would learn soon enough, Sinemet is a medicine used to ameliorate the symptoms of Parkinson's disease. It is not a cure.

As I left Dr Archer's office, my mind was spinning, unable to accept the diagnosis I'd been offered. At the time, I had a preconceived notion of Parkinson's as something aged grandparents acquire after long, fulfilling lives, not people in their prime. Someone with Parkinson's, I imagined, would already be in decline – slow, doddering, frail. I just didn't see myself that way.

Moreover, I genuinely believed I had a *running injury*. Even now, I feel defensive on this point. Like most hard-training athletes, I spent nearly as much time identifying and recovering from injuries as I spent training and competing. Being hurt became normal. My injury patterns had usually involved deficiencies on my left side, so my 'walking problem' seemed like nothing new to me. Rather than trying to accept a neurological diagnosis, I focused on all the heartache my athletic injuries had caused me over the years. Injuries forced me to miss or pull out of numerous major championships. On three occasions, I made the finals before having to withdraw.

Now, I told myself, the physical strain I'd endured to compete at the highest level of athletics was causing dysfunction that mimicked Parkinson's. Rather than let myself feel scared by Dr Archer's diagnosis, I felt bitterness toward my athletics career and the sacrifices it had required of me.

I described my feelings to Patty when I got home. There had to be a mistake, I told her, and I had no earthly intention of taking the medicine. I asked her to come outside to watch me trot down the street, to convince her that it was just a running injury, refusing to entertain even a remote possibility that my inability to run could have been the early signs of a movement disorder. Until I experienced a typical Parkinson's symptom – just a simple tremor – I would not concede.

In fact, my process of accepting my Parkinson's diagnosis had already begun.

While full denial occupied me, in some corner of my mind, I'd been storing away bits and pieces about the disease, fragments of facts gleaned as I'd gone from doctor to doctor. In the face of Dr Archer's certainty, I had new context for the spectrum of neurological pathology described to me by my sports doctor in Dublin. It wasn't lost on me that, if Dr Archer was not right, it could be much worse. I remember thinking, at least it isn't ALS.

Looking back on it, I'm inclined to forgive my stubborn unwillingness to accept what was happening to me. What I would learn about Parkinson's over the next decade would have been too overwhelming for anyone to accept all at once. While a Parkinson's diagnosis isn't a death sentence, it is a life sentence with no chance for parole.

As I would find out, Parkinson's is determined to make each day of that sentence a little worse.

Parkinson's is a movement disorder that can impair every bodily action, whether involving big muscle groups used, say, for walking, or smaller muscles recruited for fine motor skills such as brushing your teeth. Your body can become tight and rigid, making walking difficult to impossible. With repetitive actions such as brushing your teeth, you often slow down, then stall.

People with Parkinson's can suddenly freeze – in motion one moment, frozen in place the next. Freezing can have specific triggers, such as walking through a doorway. Then, of course, there are the tremors and other unwanted and uncontrollable jerks and spasms. Parkinson's can impact speech similarly, with words coming out in halting, slurred bursts and stutters. The faulty neural transmissions in people with Parkinson's can eventually prevent proper functioning of the autonomic system, which controls involuntary actions such as swallowing and saliva production.

The term 'disease' is highly descriptive of what you have to endure; the term implies the body is in a condition of dis-ease. You cannot get your body to relax. You lie on the sofa, but your hands are curled up like a t-rex. For some reason you can't get the message to them to let go, to lie in your lap like normal people. You sit on a chair, but your body is restless. A movement disorder even when you are stationary.

It's not very encouraging.

For some people, the progression of the disease is glacial; for others, the decline is rapid.

Conventional wisdom suggests that those cursed at a young age have a slower progression than those with later onsets.

To this day, I never know whether to describe the momentum of the disease as progression or regression. From Parkinson's perspective, it must be progression, proof that it is prevailing. I prefer to think of it as regression. What begins as slowness or hesitancy eventually blossoms into full-blown stiffness or cramping or the inability to swing your arms in symphony with your legs.

Of course, not content simply to mess up your walking and tooth-brushing, Parkinson's also messes with your mind, bringing restlessness and anxiety on top of frustration and anger. It's truly a smorgasbord and it can change daily.

If you or someone you know has Parkinson's, it's important to remember that the disease has a catalogue of different symptoms and that everyone's experience is a little different. As a doctor friend of mine, who also has Parkinson's, likes to say, 'Many of us have different illnesses, but we all have the same disease.'

According to the World Health Organisation, 'The cause for PD is not known but is thought to arise from a complex interaction between genetic factors and exposure to environmental factors such as pesticides, solvents and air pollution throughout life.' Recent studies, meanwhile, suggest that traumatic brain injuries, such as those from concussions, may cause a cascade of effects that eventually lead to Parkinson's. In my case, I've had little experience with chemicals other than garden weedkillers. I did, however, play rugby through five years at St Munchin's. On one occasion, I suffered a mighty skull-to-skull clash that had my head spinning like Wile E. Coyote for days.

I have never been caught up in how or why I got Parkinson's, and I have a particular lack of interest in the 'why me?' inquiry. None of those gyrations end up in a positive place. Well-intentioned people have commented, 'It will make you stronger', or 'You were chosen because you could cope.' All of that conjecture is looking backward, and I can't abrogate my past. Nothing I can do will resurrect my earlier self. My focus has to be on bending, not breaking.

I have always believed in seeing things through to the end, even when it feels you are headed for the nadir. There is always a chance that just by staying in the game, you will catch a break. Some call it luck, some call it foresight; but at the end of the day, if you hang around the goal, you will eventually score.

I experienced many tough days when I was a young athlete that taught me the benefit of persevering under difficult circumstances. Those dark days made me keenly aware that the body can endure huge amounts of hardship if the mind cares to. There were times as an athlete when nothing went smoothly, and you were still expected to perform. Back when I was racing, travel and jetlag were real challenges. The seasoned professionals cautioned against racing within three days of transatlantic travel; they figured the effects of jetlag were most extreme then. Better to wait four or five days after travel to compete.

My most poignant example of competing in harsh conditions was in Spain. The problem was getting to Spain, Seville to be precise. I heeded my predecessor's advice and planned to depart for Spain four days before competition. I even doubled down on jetlag amelioration by taking the daytime flight from New York to London. That meant that I could avoid the loss of a night's sleep, a major hurdle in jetlag attenuation.

I arrived at the airport for my flight to New York with a change of planes in Chicago. I got in line for check-in and noticed it was moving at a painfully slow pace. Each interaction was taking longer than necessary. There were raised voices, anguished looks and a malaise about the assembly of people.

I overheard a passenger say to his wife, 'We're not going to make our connection.' Then he added, 'I'll rebook us for tomorrow.'

The mood worsened as more passengers determined their fates and the flight status on the monitor changed from delayed to cancelled. Then it was my turn to discuss my travel plans. The lady was flustered and exhausted and had no interest in hearing the importance of my mission. She strongly advised that I rebook for the following day. I beseeched her to check other airlines' schedules. I was conscious that scouring the airline systems for alternate routes would eat up more time than she could spare, but I had to make that flight. Otherwise, four days would become three, and then I'd be in the death zone.

After her continued advocacy for rebooking, all of which I rebuffed,

I had a flight to St Louis connecting to Detroit. The St Louis flight was three hours later, and I had all that time to vacillate over the prudence of my decision. The following morning would begin with a 5:45am flight to JFK from Detroit. I've never been a big fan of a zero dark thirty rising and cannot understand the joy with which early risers describe their early-morning routines.

The worst-case scenario happened. I got to my room in a Detroit airport hotel at 1:30am, picked up the room phone and grumpily asked the front desk for a 4:30am wake-up call. It seemed only minutes later that the phone rang, and I heard the night receptionist whisper, 'It's your 4:30 wake-up call. Do you want me to call back to remind you?' I resisted the snooze opportunity. There wasn't a single minute to spare.

Fortunately, there were no security protocols back then. The only place I had seen security to board was in Heathrow for flights to Israel. I easily made the flight to JFK and arrived at the British Airways gate to see a fresh-looking Marcus O'Sullivan waiting on me. I had been fuelled by adrenaline, and once the anxiety of making the flight dissipated, I crashed and slept most of the way. We landed and did what all committed athletes do. We went for a training run around Bushy Park.

Then it was on to Bunter's on the high street in Teddington with our agent, Kim McDonald. After we had ordered, Kim nonchalantly mentioned the spectre of a French air traffic controller's strike the following day. It was not strange for the French labour organisations to schedule work stoppages during the busy travel season. We discussed the potential impact on our travel plans. We were flying Iberia Airlines over or around France, but definitely under French jurisdiction.

Over breakfast the following morning we tried to steel ourselves for what was certain to be an arduous day. Our flight was still officially on time, but if the French kept their word, it would shortly have a more discouraging status. We arrived at Heathrow Airport mid-morning; this was my third consecutive day of travel. Surprisingly, we were allowed to check in, but with the proviso that we should watch the monitor for flight updates. Already there was a sprinkling of delays, but it was early in the day and the French had not had their say yet.

The day dragged on and on. We rumbled from one thirty-minute delay to the next. By mid-afternoon, everyone was on edge. Gate agents were tired of questions they couldn't answer, and travellers were simply tired of not knowing. Passengers continued to arrive for later flights and the terminal was teeming with anxious people. Some flights were being allowed through, which only added to the confusion.

I kept out of the fray, sitting quietly off to the side reading a book. This slowed my heart rate and reduced stress. Sure, the race was the next day, but I had no power to influence the outcome of this strike and no amount of badgering the gate agent would be remotely helpful. Some passengers continually pestered the agents for updates. As the afternoon drew to a close, the monitors were populated with cancelled flights. One or two at first, and then scores of them in red. Ultimately most of the Iberia flights were cancelled including our flight to Seville. Then we spotted an Iberia flight to Barcelona that still had a delayed status. Miraculously, an announcement was made that boarding would begin shortly.

After three days in airports, we decided we had come too far to quit now. If we could get on the Barcelona flight that night, we would be one short flight from Seville. At least, that is what we believed. Iberia 1734 took off five hours later than scheduled and made it to Catalonia safely. We immediately made tracks for the service desk to determine the earliest time we could fly to Seville; we reasoned that if we could get there early the next morning we could rest and perhaps even sleep for a few hours and be ready to race that evening.

I greeted the agent, '*Hola, Señor.*'

He must have known I didn't speak the language based on my dreadful pronunciation and responded, 'How can I be of assistance?

It turned out he was expecting us, and he had already made arrangements for us the next morning.

'What time do you have us leaving tomorrow?'

'You depart at 8:30am,' he replied.

That sounded reasonable and meant we would surely be there mid-morning. 10:30 at the latest. But then he added, '… and you arrive at 2:30pm.'

'Pardon?' I blurted out.

It appeared the only way to get to Seville was through the capital city, Madrid. So, we had two more flights and a layover to endure. We grabbed a taxi to a nearby hotel, determined to bank as much sleep as possible. Tomorrow would be day four in airports, and there was a race at the end of the ordeal.

We woke with a sense of foreboding. We had to face another long day in three airports and at the climax of the day we had to race José Luis Gonzalez, one of the best middle-distance runners in the world over 3,000 metres. At this stage, we were numb to our circumstances and went through the day on autopilot. Finally, after eight flights and four days' travelling, we arrived at the Seville Grand hotel at 3:15pm. We had exactly three and a half hours until the gun. We were exhausted. We decided the best approach was to begin the race at the rear, find a rhythm and say a decade of the rosary. You never know, it may just click.

After a very discouraging warm-up, we toed the line with a stellar field of Spanish athletes. We had heard from Gonzalez's manager that the race would be at Spanish-record pace. All the more reason to hang back. Ironically, we didn't even ask what the record was. Fast was fast and likely too fast for us. We just wanted to do the minimum to be paid.

The race commenced, and we easily made our way to the back of the field. We practically stood still when the gun was fired and were left at the rear. The pace was hot – as was the temperature in southern Spain in June! The lively pace continued deep into the lap count as we clung to the field by a thread. I began to feel power in my fatigued legs and clawed my way up to the leading group of five with two laps remaining; made a mad dash into the lead with 150 metres to go. José Luis responded immediately and drew even at the top of the home straight. We battled to the finish line with the Spaniard getting the victory by one-hundredth of a second. He set a new Spanish record of 7:41 that evening.

Those four days were tough – just like my current condition is far less than ideal. But you have to make the best of your circumstances. You can't work with tools you don't have. The odds were slim that I would perform well. The four irksome travel days and our late arrival should have disqualified me from contention. But I minimised stress by not entertaining worst-case scenarios. The fact that a worst case ensued was not compounded by fixating on it in advance. I dealt with each setback as it arose. I didn't let the situation escalate.

This ability to compartmentalise would serve me well in adapting to the nuances of a progressive disease. I needed all my resolve to adapt to my new reality. I needed somebody to lean on.

Those first days and weeks following Dr Archer's diagnosis were rocky, and I know I wouldn't have made it without Patty. Her composure made the grim reality a bit less grim. She is hugely empathetic and extremely capable and somewhere early on in this journey, I made a conscious decision to refrain from worrying and let Patty do it for both of us. I quite simply check out of situations that cause stress.

## CHAPTER 4

# DON'T BE DISCOURAGED

After finding out I had a horrible disease and losing a job I loved dearly all within a short space of time, it might have crossed my mind that my world was collapsing. Funny enough, my life didn't fall apart – at least not right away. Force of habit carried me forward for quite a while as I played my assigned roles as well as I could.

With a few other former Alltel executives, we formed a consulting practice and secured several healthy engagements. The work kept me looking forward, gave me purpose, a sense of normalcy. It also gave me a reason to travel, which has been a big part of my life since I first left Ireland. Outside of work, I spent my days much as I always had, focused on my family, trying to enjoy time with friends, living outwardly like everything was still the same.

Early on, we secured a consulting contract to work on wireless issues for an entertainment company. The gig required me to travel to Philadelphia on a weekly basis, giving me a chance to visit my old friend Marcus O'Sullivan.

Marcus and I come from neighbouring counties in Ireland and have known each other since we were boys. Our careers in athletics are closely entwined; we were rivals, teammates and travel companions. We grew up together, saw the world together.

After athletics, Marcus continued in the perspiring arts, becoming head track coach for the Villanova Wildcats, while I made the tectonic shift to a shirt and tie job. This would be the first time those two worlds were in the same orbit. I invited Marcus into the city for a cocktail in one of those big-city, professional-type bars. He showed up wearing athletic gear, proudly adorned with a large 'V' for Villanova and comfortable-looking shoes. There was nothing comfortable about what I was wearing. Marcus was polite and easy-going with my colleagues, but I could tell he was itching to get back to the Main Line where Villanova is located.

On my next trip to Philly, Marcus invited me to his house for dinner. I took the train to Havertown, a suburb of Philadelphia. We enjoyed a great meal with his wife, Mary, reminiscing about old times, especially the contrasting experiences we'd each had at the Penn Relays. In 1981, Marcus was on the winning Villanova team (thanks to me losing a thirty-yard lead to Sydney Maree in the anchor leg of the distance medley), and in 1983, I was on the winning Arkansas team. I felt at ease with the O'Sullivans, unguarded. I even admitted to Marcus that I'd felt slighted when I wasn't offered a scholarship to Villanova. My health status? I kept that matter to myself.

The next day, Marcus called. Right away, he asked how I was doing, an edge of concern in his voice. Mary, a nurse, thought there was something up with me. 'She thinks you seemed depressed,' Marcus said.

I brushed him off, said something about the demands of my work, my busy travel schedule. I knew Marcus and Mary were on to me, but I wasn't ready to tell even my closest friends the truth.

That, I would dispense solely on a need-to-know basis.

\* \* \*

While my employment with Alltel ended shortly after the Verizon deal received the blessing of the Federal Communications Commission (FCC), my involvement with the company would continue. At the time Verizon acquired it, Alltel was doing business in thirty-four states, with nearly fourteen million subscribers.

Verizon's FCC approval to buy Alltel came with the condition that it dispose of some of those Alltel markets – what amounted to licenses, network assets, and subscribers – wherever the combined market share exceeded a certain percentage, ostensibly preventing Verizon from monopolising any of those markets.

AT&T bought a large chunk of the divested Alltel properties, but were refused approval, for similar monopoly reasons, for certain markets. Those remaining properties – only twenty-six markets, six states in total, comprising eight hundred thousand subscribers, amounting to the ninth largest wireless business in the country – continued to operate as Alltel through a trust operated by Verizon. A Boston-based company, Atlantic TeleNetworks (ATN), set out to acquire those trust markets.

Initially, ATN engaged my partners and me to get the deal across the regulatory finish line. We travelled to Washington DC to represent our client before the Department of Justice and the FCC. In the meantime, ATN began looking for someone to run the business, eventually making overtures to me and one of my partners. Both of us declined, reasoning that the markets – cut adrift, stranded – would become islands, easy for a competitor to target before the new buyer could get a foothold.

ATN, particularly the CEO, Michael Prior, didn't take no for an answer. Serendipitous circumstances caused me to listen more carefully to his overtures. That summer, while at home in Ireland, we visited a beautiful island off the Dingle Peninsula called the Great Blasket. After a choppy, twenty-minute ferry passage from a tiny pier in Dunquin, we disembarked to bright sunshine on the windward shore of the island. I smiled at the thought of a doctor making a house call out here in the dead of night.

This remote spot was once inhabited by fishermen and sheep farmers, who lived in picturesque, thatched cottages with immaculately white-washed walls. They eked out a very tough living, but eventually the lack of access to medical and educational services, not to mention social opportunities, forced the last islanders to evacuate in the 1950s. The island is well known to the Irish of my generation because an Irish-language book, *Peig*, written by an islander, Peig Sayers, tormented many of us in secondary school.

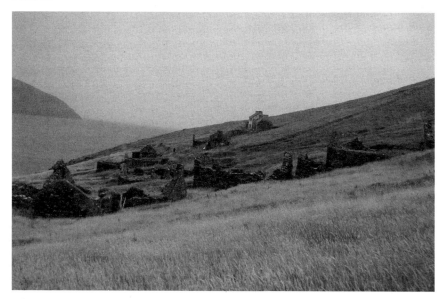

6 August 2010. Great Blasket on the afternoon Michael Prior called.

After a leisurely stroll around the island, including a brief inspection of the ruins of what once must have been a cosy cottage, my phone rang. It surprised me, I didn't see any towers, didn't think the signal would carry that far, even across water. It was Michael Prior, the CEO of ATN.

I sat down on a clump of mossy grass growing over the remnants of an ancient wall. The grass was soft like velvet and quite comfortable. I was curious how Michael had tracked me down and what he wanted, but before he said anything, I gave him a heads-up.

'I won't be able to provide much assistance,' I said. 'I'm in Ireland.'

'Where in Ireland are you?' he asked. 'My family is from County Kerry. I've been many times.'

'There's no way you've been here,' I assured him. 'I am on an island, thirty minutes off the west coast.'

'Hold on,' the voice in Boston said. 'You're not on the Blasket Islands, are you?'

I was gobsmacked.

'That's *exactly* where I am.'

Turns out, Michael's great-grandfather and his family were some of the last people evacuated from one of the Blaskets decades earlier. After battling isolation, loneliness, and dreadful weather for generations, they had made the smart call to seek greater companionship in mainland Kerry. Successive generations continued the trend of smart decision-making by emigrating to the United States, where they achieved notable business success.

What were the chances that the great-grandson of a Blasket Islander would call to offer me a CEO role at his top-ten wireless company while I'm standing on that same obscure island? The coincidence seemed too perfect to ignore. It took a few more weeks, but ultimately, Michael convinced

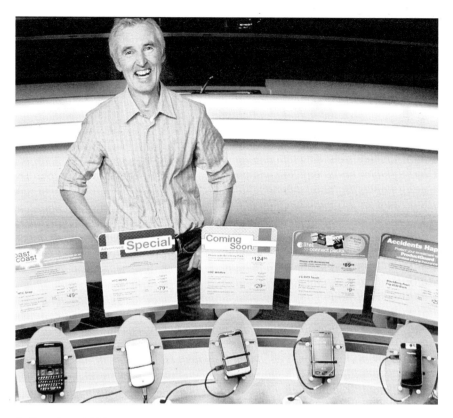

3 October 2010. CEO of Alltel Wireless (AWCC). (Photo courtesy of *Arkansas Democrat-Gazette*.)

me to join him in what became a great but arduous adventure.

First, we had to resolve an important issue for me personally, as well as for the business: where to headquarter the new company.

Patty's father, a lovely man, had recently been given a diagnosis of myelofibrosis, told he might live another three to five years. As you might guess, Patty had no intention of leaving town, and I had no intention of spending weekdays in Atlanta (where ATN proposed we locate the business) while my family remained in Little Rock. Fortunately, Michael Prior conceded that Little Rock had the advantage of a proximate workforce. We would need to hire close to a thousand people, while Verizon would be terminating hundreds of our former colleagues, making them ideal candidates for us. Michael agreed to headquarter in Little Rock.

I didn't tell Michael about my Parkinson's diagnosis. I decided that my health was a weakness, that being in charge required strength. This would be a big leadership challenge and I couldn't appear vulnerable. How do you exhort others to extreme effort if you are not capable of producing similar exertion yourself?

I did confide, however, in Wade McGill.

The first person I sought to hire, Wade was ideally suited for the fight ahead. He had that underdog approach that you often find in state school graduates, the sort of person who can make do without a lot of frills. Until we took control of the properties now held in the Verizon-controlled trust, we lacked the revenue to cover our expenses. We could spend money only when imperative, working from a makeshift office furnished with stained chairs, using 800 numbers with unsecure lines for conference calls – a practice our erstwhile partners at Verizon marvelled at, pressing to host the calls on their company's encrypted network.

Wade agreed to become our chief administrative officer, but first, there was something I had to be honest about. Somebody needed to be aware of my medical issue. In the event I needed a time out – a respite, so to speak – I needed somebody to know what was really going on. I recall our conversation vividly:

'Wade, there's something you need to know before you accept this role,' I said. 'Something only you and I can know about.'

'Sure, what is it?'

'It will require you to cover for me on occasion,' I continued.

'Anything, Frank.'

'It's hard to finesse this, so I'm just going to blurt it out: I have Parkinson's disease.'

Wade didn't immediately respond, so I jumped right in, spilling as much as I believed he could absorb: 'It's early stages, but since I was diagnosed early, it should have a slow progression profile ... and I am *perfectly* capable. I just need to pace myself.'

'No problem,' Wade said. 'Whatever you need.'

I noticed that Wade's forehead had become deeply furrowed. The corners of his mouth were quivering ever so slightly.

'Is there something wrong, Wade?' I asked.

'I've got something I ought to share, too ...' he said, '... since there may be a few times I have to disappear ... to take care of personal matters.'

'Sure. Is anything the matter?'

'My wife filed for divorce this week,' he said, flatly.

Wade is not known to elaborate, and it doesn't really matter how you get in some of these pickles; you just get on with it. He, like me, needed flexibility; we agreed to look out for each other. After some mutual consoling, Wade blurted out, 'I'd much rather be in my circumstance than in yours.'

The comment caught me off guard, but I thought about it.

Clearly, having to choose either would be an unenviable task. Better that a higher power makes those decisions. Nonetheless, I responded, 'I wouldn't swap with you.'

With all that behind us, Wade and I set about the task of staffing our new enterprise.

We had exactly a year to convert from Verizon systems to new, yet-to-be selected systems. It wouldn't be easy. Indeed, a prior purchaser of Verizon landline assets struggled to convert systems and ultimately declared bankruptcy. There were just two of us. The clock was ticking.

The greatest danger was our customer service calls were answered by a Verizon employee; and, if that employee did a poor job, our customers' option was to leave Alltel and sign up with a competitor, often Verizon itself. The same could happen in our retail stores, which were also staffed with Verizon employees. Time was clearly of the essence. The trust was losing customers or offering unsustainable pricing to retain customers – offers we couldn't afford to duplicate.

To our great frustration, the purchase agreement between ATN and Verizon precluded us from hiring former Alltel employees who were now working, albeit temporarily, for Verizon. Provisions of this nature are not unusual, but I thought ATN, conscious of the critical need for talent to convert and transition, would not have agreed to inclusion. To make matters worse, we faced severe financial penalties if we missed the conversion deadline.

To meet the deadline, we needed bodies – not just any bodies, but knowledgeable, experienced wireless professionals, at least a thousand of them. Without being able to recruit, hire, and deploy a motivated workforce quickly and efficiently, our cause was hopeless.

An obvious and immediate source of requisite talent stared us in the face: the former and soon-to-be-available Alltel employees, all of whom Verizon would ultimately terminate, anyway. They knew the systems, the networks, the business. With them, we might succeed. Without them, we had no chance.

I arranged a meeting with the person leading the Alltel transition for Verizon. Going into it, perhaps naively, I expected an acknowledgement of the difficulties we faced, followed by a reasonable adjustment to the hiring ban.

The meeting took place in the former Alltel Headquarters, by then emblazoned with the Verizon logo. As I walked into what had once been our welcoming lobby, I instantly felt uncomfortable. In the past, I'd experience just a momentary delay as a friendly security officer gave my badge a quick inspection. On this occasion, I was asked to take a seat. While I waited, I noticed how formal the environment had become. Gone was the car that Ryan Newman drove, bearing our colours, to Daytona 500 victory in 2008. We'd had to remove doors and windows to squeeze the blue Number 12 Alltel Dodge Charger into the lobby, where it sat, proudly welcoming our employees each morning.

*Oh, well,* I thought, *the car would look out-of-place here, its triumphant blue clashing against Verizon's noisy reds and blacks.* As I sat there, I felt glad to have been surplus to Verizon.

My contact arrived and introduced herself as the leader of the Alltel transition. She seemed friendly, if a bit awkward, as she tried to direct me around a building that I knew much better than she ever would.

My contact wasn't much for small talk, but she was cordial. I sensed that she was following a script, a sign that Verizon leadership had probably given her very strict instructions. When it came my turn to get down to business, I described our challenge in meeting the transition deadline without access to well-trained employees. Then I asked if she would share Verizon's employee layoff plans with me.

'You can redact names and other identifying information,' I assured her. 'I'd only ask for the area they work in and anticipated date of termination. I need the help.'

'I'm sorry,' she said, politely. 'I can't share *any* information.'

'But without the help of people familiar with the systems, we will never get it done,' I pleaded, 'and you're going to lay these people off, anyway.'

She was insouciant. 'The purchase agreement precludes you from hiring any former Alltel employee for a period of six months after severance from Verizon,' she said.

'But we only have eleven months left to complete the transition,' I countered.

The tension rose. Seated close to one another at a small office conference table, we had reached an uncomfortable stalemate. I could see the resolution in her eyes. She could probably smell the frustration on me. If she couldn't, I made it abundantly obvious when, out of the blue, my left hand began to tremor.

Did she see that? I wondered. How could she have missed it? My hands had been resting on the table, in plain sight. There was no pretending that didn't just happen. My hands were still on display. I furtively removed them, then sat on my left hand. The result was my left side began to quiver in sympathy with the misbehaving appendage.

A wave of distraction washed over me. What a time and circumstance for this to happen. I needed to concentrate, but I couldn't. The more I anguished over my unresponsive body, the more the speed of the tremor picked up. My brain tried to process the moment. Was it nerves? Although the lady had been dogmatic and immovable, she was not unpleasant. Nothing I tried could obviate the shaking; I could sense a tsunami coming. I had to get out of there before the wall of desperation hit. My only recourse was to declare the meeting over.

I left disconsolate. First, my introductory intimate experience with Parkinson's had been shared with a stranger. It would have been traumatic had it happened at home. In a contentious business meeting, it just didn't seem fair.

Second, it was evident that Verizon was never going to be a partner. A troubled conversion could only end in a mass exit of customers, looking for a new service provider with Verizon the logical alternate choice.

The enormity of the challenge was quite scary. I knew that any return ATN would make on their investment hinged on my ability to build a team that could successfully select systems and convert to them on time and on budget.

The tremor I experienced that day at Verizon forced me to categorise my business worries long enough to get focused on my persistent health issue. As usual, I began by wondering if the tremor might have been merely a natural response to the acrimonious nature of the meeting. The alternative possibility – that Dr Archer was right – had been gaining traction with me, however. As I'd had to do with Wade McGill a few weeks earlier, I found myself accepting my PD diagnosis when called upon, in a professional context, to plan responsibly for the future.

When I got home that night, I told Patty that I would try the Sinemet, as Dr Archer had advised.

Then, I decided to take Dr Archer's other suggestion: we would also seek a second opinion. We scheduled an appointment with a Parkinson's specialist at an out of state movement disorder clinic.

The decision to seek a second opinion made sense. It was the rational thing to do – like getting multiple quotes when bidding a job. Still, I felt my emotions kick in, anxiously wanting a good second opinion, hoping against hope. After a prolonged wait in a crowded waiting room, with only a few tattered *PEOPLE* magazines as distraction, we were ushered to an examination room, where we began a second round of waiting.

Eventually, a nurse arrived to take my vitals, which gave the appearance the appointment had begun. After the nurse departed, we began round two and hour two of the waiting game. After that, a young Czech doctor entered to take my detailed history. What were my symptoms? When was the first symptom? Who had I seen about the problem?

I leaned toward Patty and whispered, 'I don't understand what we are doing. Shouldn't the doctor evaluate me independently?'

'Surely he knows what he is doing?' Patty admonished, a dig in my side for my trouble.

We were with the young Czech doctor for ages; I would guess at least forty-five minutes. He was very pleasant, but we came all this distance to see the specialist, highly touted as 'the Man' in Parkinson's.

At last, he arrived, all business, matter of fact, bordering on brusque. He perused the notes that the associate had taken and performed the standard tests I'd already been through. Upon completion, he pronounced that my doctor in Little Rock was right on the money. He spent all of four or five minutes with us before hurrying off to the next poor soul.

I didn't have much time to process this second opinion. The doctor's busy schedule had put us in real danger of missing our flight home. Scrambling to arrange a taxi, we left the office in a rush, wondering how someone so efficient could be that far behind schedule. I would consider the latest Parkinson's feedback when I got back to the quiet of our home. We made the flight by the skin of our teeth. Patty and I played gin rummy on the plane – anything to avoid discussing the hurried doctor's opinion. As it turned out, Patty and I didn't discuss the subject much at all that night. There was no new information to consider, and the topic was exhausting. We left it for the next day.

* * *

I found further distraction as I continued staffing my new undertaking. I badly needed a systems expert to lead us through the complexities of the conversion. The right person needed remarkable project management skills, had to be tough and brave enough to join our quixotic quest while the rest of the telecom world was betting against us. I knew just such a person; we had been in many a dogfight together at the old Alltel. Unlike me, he was retained by Verizon, at least for the meantime. Verizon had implied that he had a future with them, but everyone knew he'd become dispensable.

Lewis Langston had a reputation for being pugnacious and prickly. It wasn't his fault; his role frequently required him to be the bad guy. I knew Lewis was determined to soften his edges in the spirit of self-improvement, but I wasn't so sure this was the environment to change his approach. Some tough roles require tough individuals.

I needed Lewis, but I had to gauge his interest. We were good friends and could not be prohibited from interacting; I knew one place I could casually run into him.

The purchase agreement between ATN and Verizon expressly prohibited the hiring of former employees for six months after Verizon terminated their employment. I had to gamble that Verizon's insistence on its anti-hire provision would be perceived as an undue restriction on workers in Arkansas, a right-to-work state. I just needed Lewis to show interest in switching horses.

Lewis is an avid bike rider, and I knew his likely route. I could still ride, so I set out to casually run into Lewis on the river trail. There was a catch:

I could ride in a straight line and, under extreme pressure, maybe manage a wide sweeping turn, a bit like an eighteen-wheeler making a ninety-degree turn. I needed a long, mostly straight road, with little traffic to interfere with my wide, clumsy turns. I knew the perfect spot on the far side of the river, where the road dead ends in a park. I drove over to the park, unloaded my bike and nonchalantly rode back and forth until Lewis appeared in the distance. I gathered myself and pedalled confidently toward my unsuspecting friend.

'Lewis?' I said, grabbing my brakes and sounding downright surprised to see him. 'I didn't know you rode in cold weather!'

Based on the gossip he'd been hearing about my health, Lewis probably wasn't expecting to see me out riding, but his first concern was my categorisation of him as a fair-weather rider.

As we pulled to the side of the road, he declared, 'I ride all year ever since I got the new all-carbon bike. And what the devil are you doing on a road bike?'

'I just had to get out …' I said, '… and I thought I might run into you.'

Standing over our bikes by the side of the road, we immediately began talking about the impending conversion. Lewis listened intently as I brought him quickly up to speed. He soon recognised that our backs were against the wall. I moaned on about the lack of cooperation I was getting from Verizon, but I could already see the wheels turning. I finished my casual, between-you-and-me update and added, 'We need an accomplished IT executive. If you know a suitable candidate, please pass on their contact info.'

Lewis took a moment, maybe two.

'Why don't I join you?' he said.

It was just that simple. Lewis had declared his interest in joining us. In that moment we both understood the conversation was over. There would be no further contact between us until he gave Verizon his notice.

Then he rode off without another word.

## CHAPTER 5

# KEEP YOUR WORD

**M**y contentment didn't last long – three weeks, to be exact. Once Verizon discovered that Lewis had joined us, they quickly filed a lawsuit in federal court in both Arkansas and New York. The lawsuit listed Lewis as the defendant. Naturally we would defend Lewis, but we also had to challenge the killer blow a Verizon victory would have on our capacity to hire staff. We had chosen Little Rock as headquarters for this new enterprise because of access to all this talent, talent that would be looking for work shortly. We couldn't let Verizon snatch defeat from the jaws of victory.

The cause of action claimed that Lewis, as a senior executive, had access to confidential and proprietary information about Verizon systems and that he couldn't be trusted to abide by his confidentiality agreement, which would require him to recuse himself from any negotiations concerning transition services.

Verizon sought an injunction to prevent Lewis from joining us. The case was heard in the new federal court building and there was tight security as we entered. We made our way to the courtroom and waited for the entrance of Judge Moody, who had been appointed to the federal bench by President Clinton. Judge Moody was older now but still imperturbable. He had an imposing presence. When the heavy wooden door creaked open, he was accompanied by his faithful companion, a retriever named Rosie. The formality of his black gown was juxtaposed with the leash-less Labrador. They took a seat. The judge in a high-back leather chair that reclined a little too far. The lab equally comfortable on the hardwood floor of the podium.

The courtroom was called to order and opening statements began. It was quickly evident that the Verizon team was grasping. Wade testified that any sales representative would be more capable of navigating a billing system or customer service desktop than Lewis. Lewis ultimately revealed that he didn't even have a billing system authorisation.

I testified before the court for around thirty minutes. Most of my anxiety surrounded the timing of my medication. If I timed it right, I would have two hours where I felt well enough to offer lucid testimony. If I got it wrong, it could be embarrassing. I couldn't control the tempo of the trial. I knew the order witnesses would be called and made my best guess when to dose. Fortunately, I was sworn in at a time that allowed me to be cogent for the duration I was on the stand.

We stressed the alleged effort to lessen employment opportunities for the former Alltel employees who would be and were being laid off by Verizon. We reaffirmed our commitment to work with them on coordinating a hiring process. Just give us a timeline for termination, and we will work within those constraints.

Judge Moody agreed with us, declaring in his opinion, 'The court is also cognisant of the chilling effect an injunction would have on Verizon employees who, in the face of an insecure job future, are examining the job market in Arkansas.'

Furthermore, he whole-heartedly rejected the contention that Lewis would not honour his severance agreement when he wrote, Verizon had 'failed to prove that Langston's new job posed a real and immediate threat to its trade secrets.'

Our lawyers cited the federal opinion from Arkansas in the New York court and that case was dismissed. We agreed that Verizon would share termination timelines by work discipline, and we could then recruit, but not before.

This victory was a massive relief to me. If we had lost Lewis, he would be out of work. Plus, we would be precluded from hiring former Alltel employees, the very reason we chose Little Rock. Foremost in my mind was the commitment I made to Michael. I assured him we'd get the job done.

* * *

I had made a few promises in the past; the most significant of which was one I made to my father back in 1976. It was late May and St Munchin's College never looked better. Perched on a nothing hill on the banks of the curving River Shannon, the school had just enough elevation to command a view over Ireland's longest river. On this clear day you could see Moylussa, the highest point in County Clare, way in the distance. The groundskeepers took advantage of a rare dry morning to take the top couple of inches off the playing fields, and the smell of freshly mowed grass lingered in the air. It wasn't necessarily hot, but in the direct sun, particularly behind a glass window, we could feel the rays warming our faces as we cleared out our cubicles.

My younger brother, Brendan, and I were especially excited that our father was expected to pick us up. He had been away in the UK the previous few times we had been home and undoubtedly would have some trinket for each of us from his travels. My last gift was a little sought after Tranmere Rovers cap that he brought back from a weekend at the Cheltenham Racing festival. It didn't matter that it wasn't nearby Liverpool or Everton. It was from my dad.

My father was gregarious and fun. He drank socially, played cards, and even smoked the odd Henri Wintermans cigar. He once played the big drum in the Tulla Céilí Band when he was younger. He seemed to know everyone and was keenly interested in local politics. He brought us to election counts as observers late into the night. His business was going well, and he enjoyed the benefits of its success. He spent his growing leisure time horse racing, dog racing and watching hurling and football matches. He even took us to the Market's Field and Thomond Park to watch the English sports soccer and rugby. He loved competition of any kind.

He nurtured our competitive tendencies, frequently pitting my brother and me against each other. His favourite challenge was a run to the local corner shop. It began with him or my mother requiring something, and the ploy was simple. 'Francis, do you think you can make it to Walsh's and back for a loaf of bread in less than two minutes?' he would ask.

'I can, Dad!' my brother Brendan would interrupt before I could answer.

Some minor hand-to-hand combat would then ensue between Brendan and me as I exclaimed, 'He asked *me*, not you!'

These disputes were solved in predictable fashion. 'Francis will get the bread and then Brendan will get the newspaper. I'll time you both separately.'

After lodging a complaint about the difficulty of transporting a sliced pan versus the *Limerick Leader*, the contest would begin. The course had several hazards. First, you had to bound up and over a ladder that traversed a hedge separating our yard from the Walshes' who were great friends and the shop's proprietors. Next you navigated the narrow pathways through the vegetable garden while avoiding the glasshouses. Then you undid the latch on the outside of the back yard gate. This was not easily done as you had to reach over the gate to do so. After carefully dodging any cars in the drive, you were only a 180-degree turn on the main Ennis Road from the destination. The Ennis Road is one of the busiest streets in Limerick. You had the width of footpath to safely make the corner, enter the store, put the bread on our account and then repeat the journey home.

The last obstacle on the return trip was daunting. On the Walsh side, the ground was higher, and you could easily make the top of the ladder with one bound, but were you brave or desperate enough to hurdle it? The landing was tricky. Finally, you burst through the back door to hear my father counting a minute: fifty-two, fifty-three, fifty-four ... These races usually ended in a tie. It took us a while to figure out the charade, but we kept participating. It's a bit like admitting you don't believe in Santa Claus; you're afraid the gift-giving will cease. In this instance, the concern was continuous access to Cadbury's Dairy Milk chocolate and our father's attention.

Those races to the shops with my brother were the first signs that I had a proclivity for racing. I had suspected I was fast. As an underage footballer, I was accustomed to getting in the first team; selectors knew I would run till I dropped. I was well aware that I hadn't developed real dribbling skills, I merely pushed the ball beyond the opposing player and caught up with it faster than he could.

The first real indicator that I was fast was at St Munchin's. Each night after dinner there was about a thirty-five-minute recreational period before three hours of study hall. While daylight savings lasted, before the long lonesome, dark winter nights, boarders played soccer on the big yard, or on one of two tennis courts, or played handball in one of four alleys. There were a few prized indoor attractions, such as a snooker table and a foosball table. With roughly two hundred poor souls in lockdown there were clearly not enough outlets for everyone to enjoy. A tradition had been developed to assign the limited resources. Not a rotation system, as would have been most equitable, but a less elegant 'winner takes all' approach. The first student to touch the desired piece of ground would secure rights for his group. This meant the older or stronger upperclassmen had the advantage and rarely did you see younger kids playing, especially on the big yard.

Dinner always began and ended with grace. The dean rose at the front of the refectory, under the crucifix, and just to the left of the double-wide exit doors he had opened as the cue to stand. During the meal, we sat ten to a table, and there were over twenty tables. It was noisy and loud at the best of times, but as dinner closed it got quiet and suspenseful. While most students stood for the prayer at their appointed seats, those tasked with acquiring recreational space began to assemble around the newly opened doors. By the time the priest had given thanks for the less than adequate meal, there was a proper crowd waiting for the signal, the last word of the sign of the cross '… and the Holy Ghost, AMEN'. The first syllable was set and the second was go.

The bigger kids used their size to prevent the smaller, nimbler kids from getting a toe on the line. The smaller trying to squeeze between the massive waists of intimidating rugby players. One eye on the priest and one on the open door. There were false starts, particularly if the dean purposely paused before the Amen, like Messi taking a penalty kick. Any false start was punished by elimination, you were ignominiously sent back to your table. You and your buddies would be watching others play that evening.

Finally, 'Amen' was heard and there was a clatter of chairs, heavily discarded against the wall, and the sound of someone who had taken an elbow in the solar plexus, gasping for air. The initial run was about forty metres long, terminated into the study-hall wall and required a high-speed ninety-degree turn. Inevitably, someone misjudged his approach or received an inopportune push in the back and ended up spattered against the wall. Seasoned runners knew it was imperative and even prudent to let the older kids dominate this first stretch, avoid calamity and surge in the wider middle sector, which was over double the distance. Then one more ninety-degree turn – this time without an impenetrable wall as a back stop – and you had twenty metres remaining to the exit to the playing fields.

Some of the older boarders noticed that I was frequently in the mix at that second pivotal turn. I was excited to be recognised by upperclassmen, but uncertain how that would work. Did I have to play with them too? There was no rule book to refer to except tradition, which had been handed down by previous students. Tradition was under attack.

I, a mere fourteen-year-old, agreed to represent a group of seniors who had the misfortune of regularly missing out on the big yard. The pressure was on. I ran cleverly, held back through the initial turn and surged in the middle longer section and was first to the yard. The seniors were delighted and engaged me similarly the following week. Once again, I deployed the same tactics and was first to the exit and was certain to be the first to touch the yard. A few metres before I made the final and all-important step, I heard and felt an object whizz past my left ear. Then I saw a small ball bounce once, then twice, three times on the yard in front of me … Immediately, before I made my imprint of the surface, I heard celebration from someone behind me.

This fella now claimed that *he* had won. Knowing that only the two of us were witness, I complained, 'You threw a ball. I was first to step on the yard.'

Others started to arrive, and a crowd surrounded both of us. Quickly, it became obvious that the previous week's losing group had interpreted the rules not unlike my benefactors had done the previous week. An almighty brouhaha broke out between the groups. The claimants asserted that there was nothing saying *what* had to touch. If the rubber sole of a shoe was good enough, why not the rubber surface of a ball?

After a heated discussion, it was wisely decided to revert to the original interpretation of the tradition, no more designees and no more ball-throwing. I was no longer needed. The only obligation I felt was when winter rolled round and we raced for radiators to huddle around just to stay warm. The boarding school with tall ceilings and draughty single-glazed windows was forever cold and radiators were coveted for their instant warmth. We followed the same routine. First to touch got to hang on to that radiator for half an hour and warm himself and a few pals before we spent three hours of inactivity in the study hall.

I would not be exposed again to representing others until running on relay teams for Irish schoolboys at the FISEC games (the International Sports Federation for Catholic Schools) and in one of the many relay carnivals in college. Meanwhile, I had been recognised by my peers as one of the fastest in our school. I could build on that.

At the end of the 1976 school year, as we packed up for summer break, the dormitory was alive with excitement. There was a definite buzz among the students. Today we would be dismissed for the summer holidays.

Dismissal would be at noon, there was no elaborate event or celebration to mark the occasion, no Top Student award, and no most likely category awards. You were dismissed and simply left. A large brass bell signalled schedule changes throughout the day. It was a relic from the old campus which dated back to the school's founding in 1776. The bell looked at least that age. It took two hands to ring, and it generated an impressive screeching noise. It could be heard throughout the huge building and even out on the sports fields. There were multiple patterns to convey different alerts, but on the last day the bell just rang. Immediately, the day pupils were gone, seemingly vanished into thin air.

Boarders, on the other hand, had a rigorous protocol to follow. Beds had to be stripped, lockers cleaned out, clothes packed. We were under strict orders to leave things neat and tidy. Most did just enough to pass the checkout inspection. We didn't allow the delay to dampen our enthusiasm. We were excited to get home after a full term away. We would sleep in, enjoy edible meals, and hang out with family and neighbourhood friends. Not that boarding school is entirely miserable, but by year end you have had your fill of the daily grind, which begins with mass at 6:30, followed by study hall, all before breakfast.

Amidst all the preparation to depart, I was summoned to the President's office by the Prefect.

'Francis O'Mara, Fr MacNamee wants to see you in his office.'

'Now?' I replied curtly, as I was making progress cleaning my cubicle.

The Prefect who was interrupted from his studies to fetch me was in an obdurate state of mind.

'Yes, O'Mara. Right now.'

The President, Fr MacNamee, was a wonderful older man who I knew well from his interest in athletics. It surprised me when I saw my brother

Brendan waiting on my arrival. Fr McNamee greeted us formally. He instructed us to sit and informed us that our father had suffered a heart attack. He had been taken by ambulance to the Regional Hospital and was in the intensive care unit.

Like most young boys, we loved our dad, and we struggled to make sense of the news. Shock set in, and we just sat there and stared at the President.

My first thought was, *Mom will come get us, and she'll explain everything.* But no, the Dean said, 'Your mother is at the hospital, and a neighbour and shopkeeper, Willie Walsh, will pick you up.'

I replied calmly. 'Will we come back to get our belongings after we go to the hospital?'

His response surprised me. 'You're not going to the hospital. Mr Walsh is taking you home.'

'But why not?' I exclaimed.

'You're too young to visit a patient in an ICU,' was the concise response I received.

For some reason, in those days fifteen-year-olds were not allowed in the intensive care units of hospitals. I couldn't understand that rule. Perhaps it was related to the lack of private rooms with all the cardiac patients piled into a single ward. You don't want noisy kids milling around people who are in real danger of a catastrophic cardiac event. I couldn't visit my father, but my mother suggested each of us write him a letter. I vowed to do just that. Write and tell him how important he was to me.

It was a typical teenage letter. I began with some trivial fare about another futile trip to an athletics event in Dublin. I related where we stopped on the way home, who drove and what we had eaten. I had just finished third or fourth in the Irish Schools Athletics Championships, comprehensively beaten in the Intermediate 1,500 metres. The lack of success was bewildering to me and a cause of growing frustration. I had been close on many occasions. The streak of average performances began when I finished third in the all-Ireland under-elevens. Here I was four years later, and I had not managed to taste victory. I knew my father was equally baffled by my inability to reach the top of the podium, which only served to heighten my woe.

I took a deep breath and promised my father I would win the Intermediate Schools title the following year. This was a brazen move by my standards, but I hoped this promise would encourage him to get well so that he

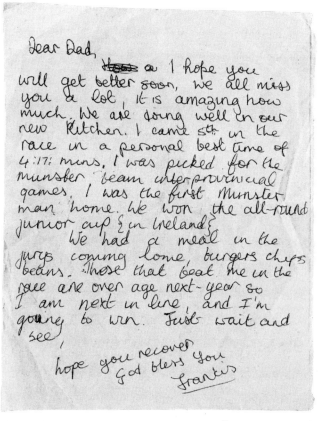

6 June 1976. A fifteen-year-old's promise, 'I'm going to win. Just wait and see.'

could witness my success for himself. In that moment, I didn't understand the gravity of that promise, let alone the effort required to honour it. I merely intended to provide an incentive for my father to live. I wanted to contribute to the solution. How did we get Dad back home?

There wasn't much in the tangible evidence category when I enquired how he was doing, although reports from the adults who could visit him were encouraging. The ICU merely seemed to provide a greater degree of observation. There were no stents placed and no bypass performed. My father was monitored, for fear of a second – often fatal – heart attack. That is precisely what happened. My father died a week later never having left that ward.

My mother had just returned from visiting him in the hospital and declared that he was doing well. No sooner had she spoken than the phone rang.

My uncle answered and said, 'Cissie, it's for you. It's the Regional Hospital.'

My mother sprang to the phone and replied, 'This is Mary O'Mara. Is something the matter?'

Then there was crying. Crying that seemed to last for years. My uncle who answered the phone took over the call as my mom collapsed into his arms. Between sobs she whispered to me, 'Your beautiful father is gone.'

That is about as lucid as she would be for years. I went outside and cried hopelessly.

It is beyond a shame. These days, doctors would put in a couple of stents, and my father would be back at the Mallow Races or an evening meeting at Limerick Junction within a week. Sadly, it turned out my schoolboy scrawl was the last communication I ever had with him.

He was only sixty-four years old, and we carried the same name. To avoid confusion, I was referred to as Francis, a name I could barely abide. It felt too feminine to me. The dislike originated in primary school when another kid referred to me as 'Lady Frances.' Now there was no 'e' in the male version, but that distinction was lost on nine-year-olds. Within days of my father's passing, I declared my intention to be referred to as the more mature Frank.

Time obviates the feeling of loss. At least, that is what people would say. I guess the grieving somehow comes to an end, but the sense of loss never does. I still miss my dad to this day. I wish my wife and kids had known him. They only see a balding man in a black and white picture on a shelf. The grieving process for me was entangled with this commitment I had made. I could have shrugged it off as idle words merely intended to fill a page and complete a mother's request. Who would hold me accountable in the first place? I ruminated on my personal best of 4:14 and how far behind the leading runners I was. In a moment of clarity, I decided to embrace the commitment as a shared bond between father and son. I could honour my father's memory by winning for him. The effort would consume me for an entire year.

This quest to become the 1977 Irish Schools 1,500-metre champion was officially on. To be successful everything needed to be taken up two or three notches. My coach suggested a morning session twice a week at 6am, Mondays longer hill repeats and Wednesdays a shorter version. There was power in sacrifice. Twice a week I got up early to do hill work on the Mill Road behind St Munchin's. At 5:30, my tiny alarm sounded in my dormitory cubicle, and I quietly rose and slinked along the cold ceramic floors. The long wide halls were ink-dark without the occasional illumination emitted by modern exit or emergency signs. Then I made my way to the dungeon-like dressing rooms in the basement to put on my running gear. It was still pitch dark when I met up with my coach and a few other determined souls.

The dormitory held seventy kids, and we all slept within arm's length of each other. So I kept the alarm under my pillow with one hand in close proximity. The clock vibrated when it rang, and I used the vibration to locate the off button before the second ring. If I failed to shut it off on the first ring, I risked waking somebody. Sleep was a valued commodity at boarding school. We had prayer in the chapel each night from 10:15 to 10:30. Lights out in each dormitory was twenty minutes later. We were back in church for morning mass at 6:30 the next day.

I kept up this routine for an entire year. I pushed everything to the maximum. I did circuit training in the gym. I lifted weights. I set records on training runs, but the critical factor in my new mindset was the early morning sessions. They set the tone for the entire year. Without them, what would be the distinction between me and my competitors? Instead of envying my sleeping dorm mates, I viewed them as surrogates for my competition. While they were sleeping, I was working.

The traditional first test of the athletics season was the North Munster Schools Championships, and I was determined to set the proper tone for the season. I was prepared both physically and mentally. To a spectator the journey was just beginning, but I had been on this crusade for over nine months. I was concerned that the emotional journey may have caused excessive exuberance, so I adapted my race plan to accommodate the pent-up fire. My usual tactic had been to start well, then drift back to around middle pack, truthfully even further back, launch a desperate last-minute sprint and hopefully claw my way back to the front.

There was no such indecision in 1977. My determination needed a release. I went straight to the front, applied as much early pressure as possible and hung on for all I was worth. This newly discovered resolve may have appeared as self-confidence, but it was simply raw determination. I handily won the 1,500 metres in a time of 4:08. I cut six seconds off my previous best in my first run of the season. The Munster Schools were next and were expected to provide a sterner test. I deployed the same tactics yielding a similar victory with a further seven-second improvement to my best. I reduced my personal record to 4:01 from 4:14 in two weeks. I ran with the same conviction in the 800 metres at both championships and was rewarded with wins in each.

I had enjoyed victory at previous Munster Schools Championships; it was at the national level that I came undone. The Irish Schools Athletics Championships are the largest theatre in underage athletics in Ireland. They are contested by competitors from all thirty-two counties and are the platform on which careers are constructed (or more commonly shattered). The enormity of the task was not lost on me. After all, I had failed at this juncture in the past. Added to the intensity, the championships were held on my home track at Plassey where my father would certainly have been in his customary spot. My mother would be there in his place. She was a nervous observer more likely to avert her eyes at a critical moment than to shout encouragement.

There are two major conflicting emotions before all races — a clash between nerves and desire.

Hopefully, desire wins. In this instance, although nerves were at an all-time high, they never really had a chance. I was driven by a year-old promise. Naturally, it was a tremendous bonus to not have to worry about tactics. They were set in stone. I was committed to front running. I knew how the race would begin, and I was determined to dictate how it would finish.

I decided not to race the 800 metres and put all my energies into the 1,500 metres. This allowed me to remain at St Munchin's, just five miles away, until the last minute. I arrived an hour before my race and was anxious, but not intimidated when I stood on the starting line. I imagined my father standing trackside with his peaked cap tilted a little sideways. I resolved at that moment that nobody would prevent me from fulfilling my obligation. I charged into the lead from the gun and sprinted to the curve. The first lap took fifty-nine seconds, sub-four-minute mile pace. Surely no sixteen-year-old could sustain that sort of early pressure? The question was, could I? I managed to survive my early exuberance and won by a full straight in a new personal best of 3:58.2. That time was a new Irish Schools record by 4.1 seconds and survived as the National Record for over thirty years. There was immediate joy followed by an instant release of pressure. I was finally an all-Ireland champion, but to this day the memory is bittersweet. It is impossible to untangle the sadness from the success.

When my mother passed away in 2013, we found the letter I had written among her possessions, and upon reading it, my recollection was immediate and vivid. Not especially of that day in Plassey, but of the complete process. A year-long mission to honour my deceased father, a year of grieving. My mother often told me that my father gave a little wry smile when he read the letter, but she never revealed that she secured it. That teenage writing turned out to be a watershed moment in my life. I felt an enormous bond with my father throughout the year, and in the process, I found my identity and a purpose.

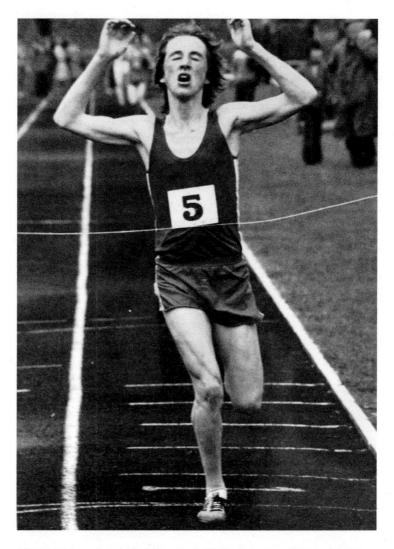

June 1977. Wining the Irish Schools 1,500m by a convincing margin.

Later that summer, I managed a further six-second improvement to end the season with a best of 3:52. A full twenty-two second improvement in one year. Enough reason to continue the approach that reaped such a generous reward. While I maintained the same application and work effort, I strangely discarded the successful race day tactics. After that season, I went back to the standard sit and kick tactics. Perhaps I associated front running with my father and the grieving process or perhaps, not having that one special person to impress, I simply was not as obsessively compelled. It is the only year I ran from the front in a competitive race. In truth, I ran scared because I was too frightened to disappoint. I had a promise to fulfil.

\* \* \*

When I accepted the stewardship of AWCC, I thought of the young boy I was then, and of that year of hard training and commitment to a goal. Now I was faced with another huge promise, the one I'd made to Michael Prior. A commitment that would take multiple years to honour and one that would require a Herculean effort. My health struggles would compound the degree of difficulty. I had serious doubts about my ability to stay focused on the task, given the distractions of the now uncontrollable shaking on my left side. The more I pushed, the angrier the disease became. But I was determined to deliver. This wasn't a particularly large company; it had almost a million customers and a billion dollars in revenue. But I realised that it would likely be my only opportunity to be a CEO. It would be a complete test of our resolve. We had to operate a business and build a second company concurrently. Then swap customers from one business to another in mid-flight. With three or four employees and a ticking clock, a promise to fulfil indeed.

## CHAPTER 6

# GREAT RESULTS REQUIRE GREAT RISK

I had seen older people with a tremor before and I always imagined any discomfort they may have felt was isolated to that quaking appendage. I was wrong. The shaking itself at times can be limited to just a hand or it can spread like a contagion. At the very least, it is an enormous distraction. You simply cannot concentrate because the shaking dominates and takes control.

You know everyone can see your tremor, which further compounds your anxiety. You try your very best to shut it down, but you simply can't. The distraction transforms into confusion and eventually paralysis. You realise someone is talking, perhaps even to you, but you don't have the where-withal to engage. Decision-making is impossible.

Other times my entire body becomes tense, as if on the starting line waiting on the gun. You try to relax, but your body will not heed the command. How ironic that a disease that restricts movement cannot complete its supposed mission and shut down entirely. It will not allow you peace of any sort. The brain will not permit you to find a comfortable position for your arms. You feel pressure on your chest as if you are about to suffer a panic attack. I scan my to-do list and reassign any outstanding tasks to another time. Neither activity provides any relief. The enormous weight still sits uneasily on my chest.

All I can do is concentrate on my breathing. I try to settle my arms, but they are tense and heavy. I decide to put them in my pockets to quench the restlessness, but it takes one to get the other in, and I can't seem to get the second in. I take a hand back out and drape it over the arm rest. Next, I try sitting on them. If I could only concentrate on my breath ... breathe in, breathe out, breathe, in breathe out. Somehow you must get inside your body and calm the system from within.

One day as I stared at my misbehaving hand, I noticed an odd phenomenon. When I moved my hand, let's say to turn a page, the shaking ceased. It was then I realised the absence of a tremor when my hand is active. A Parkinson's tremor typically exists when the muscles are inactive. The very thought of moving your arm can cause the shaking to cease. The trick is to bifurcate the typical command into 'Get ready' and 'Go'. You get ready, but you don't go, initiate, but don't engage. The process happens in microseconds, so it takes real practice and concentration. This manoeuvre has a short shelf life. It seems the brain recognises it has been hacked and abnormal service is reinstated.

Parkinson's is caused by deterioration of cells in the basal ganglia area of the brain that produce the neurotransmitter dopamine. Nobody knows for certain what causes the destruction of these critical cells. As dopamine production is compromised, critical signalling paths are damaged or destroyed, limiting your ability to control your muscles. A typical presentation features a tremor, but these can be accompanied by cramping, rigidity and freezing.

No muscle group is denied participation. The muscles of the mouth can fail to respond to commands, jeopardising your speech, muscles in the feet curl up and cramp, even your bowel movements are compromised.

Depression is also prevalent among Parkinson's sufferers. There is an abundance of evidence that the disease itself is a contributor to depression and anxiety, due to changes in brain chemistry – the reduction of dopamine, a neurotransmitter that prevents your brain from exercising control. The same pathways that create dopamine in the brain also create the brain chemical serotonin, which regulates mood, appetite, and sleep. Scientists think that the effect of Parkinson's on serotonin, as well as other brain chemicals that support mood, is responsible for symptoms of depression and anxiety. Dopamine is also part of the brain's reward system that helps you feel pleasure and happiness. So, Parkinson's has the power not only to prevent you doing what you love, but the power to prevent you loving what you do.

The primary treatment for Parkinson's is artificial dopamine marketed in the USA under the brand name Sinemet; this is what I was prescribed by Dr Archer at the very start of my Parkinson's journey. A beginner's dose is three or four pills of 100mg per day, and it is effective especially in the early days. The treatment outcome is much different than you are accustomed to with a garden-variety antibiotic, the benefits of which accrue over time, each subsequent pill layering on an extra degree of improvement. We are programmed to believe that taking medicine remedies an ailment. Not so with Parkinson's, instead every Sinemet dose starts a new race. Once the effect wears off, you are back at the starting line every three or four hours. Sinemet merely helps you survive until the next dose.

Each pill has an efficacy window. After consumption, there is a period of absorption as the pill dissolves into the blood stream before reaching peak levels and wearing off. There is a trough between each cycle when the initial dose loses usefulness, and the next dose is not yet productive. This is referred to as an 'Off Period'.

Managing Off Periods became the battle within the war. The number of Off Periods is determined by the number of daily doses. If you take four doses there are five of these periods to manage, beginning and end of each day and the three troughs within the day. The more advanced the Parkinson's, the more troublesome the Off Periods. I dread these Off Periods. When one is imminent, I invariably tighten up. Here we go again. Imagine, if every time a cowboy rode his steed, he had to break it in. You have five breaking sessions daily and the horse is just as unruly the fifth time.

In anticipation, everything is put on hold. I have to knuckle down for however long it takes to survive the battle. I am distracted. I can't make decisions. This is the time to grin and bear it. When I was younger – sorry, before Parkinson's – I had to be involved in every household decision. These days I have little interest in the mundane, and at times would allow a Nigerian prince access to my bank account. It has been decided in our house that I should not answer the phone for fear I fall for a timeshare scheme.

Everyone around you realises you are out of commission for a while, and they work around you.

They may ask if it's time for a little yellow pill, but by and large they are observers. You take the Sinemet and bear down. A sense of euphoria announces the end of an Off Period as the Sinemet advances like waves on a beach, a steady infusion of artificial dopamine.

My particular brand had developed into full body tremoring. Almost seizure-like. It was akin to extreme restless leg syndrome, but shared with all the limbs and torso. I could predict when an attack was imminent from watching the time, but I could also sense the tsunami. My wonderful assistant, a thoughtful and caring person named Lile Harbison, and I collaborated to deal with this predicament at work. I alerted her to any occurrence and she interjected and informed whatever group I was meeting with that I had another matter that needed attention. Then she locked my office door while I lay on the floor and thrashed it out, taking deep and long breaths to quieten my noisy body. We put an opaque film on the glass interior walls so nobody could see me writhing on the floor. Without her, I could not have survived. We coordinated my meetings to avoid exposing others to the real me. We kept him behind closed doors.

Part of my anxiety was honestly the embarrassment of being seen in that condition. You want to feel normal, but instead the shaking robs you of your dignity. It renders you an object of wild curiosity, even derision. I longed to blend in, but that was impossible, particularly at work. I had to hide. I could not expose others to this calamity. I also didn't want others to worry about me. There was nothing they could do but make a fuss.

As time shoved on, the Off Periods became more irksome and persistent. So, I needed more privacy to ride out the storm. We had rented a four-storey building in west Little Rock. The arrangement allowed us to expand into the space as our employee numbers grew. The floor beneath mine was unoccupied, and I used it as a refuge. I needed real privacy and quiet to deal with the sideshow. I made that floor my triage centre. When I sensed a pending Off Period, I made straight for the stairwell to that floor. There was no electricity, and it was dark on the floor. It was formerly a call centre and was wide open office space with the exception of a few interior supervisor offices with glass panels to illuminate the space with whatever light was available. There were two smaller and odd-looking rooms. Neither had windows, just four sheet-rock walls, about six feet square. These rooms were referred to as 'comfort rooms' in the call centre trade, a place for nursing mothers or a stressed-out rep who needed some quiet time. A perfect location for my escapade.

This room was close to perfect with the exception of the awful worn carpet tile floor and its size. I had to lie diagonally to fit. I needed a no stimulation environment, no light, no noise. This was as much as I could hope for. After I got accustomed to the unforgiving hard floor, I began the process of trying to relax. I had to hold out until the next pill kicked in. I tried to muzzle the shaking. I would gain control for a while, then lose it again. It was a tug of war between my quivering body and my brain. If I could focus on the breath and ignore my body, I could break the shaking. It takes a lot of concentration when your body is in such torment. In time, I would prevail or, more likely, the Sinemet would finally reach the blood stream. Either way, any victory was temporary. I would be back in around three hours to repeat the performance.

Occasionally people would venture onto the floor to make a sensitive personal call, but they invariably stood by a window. There were a couple of conversations I wish I had not overheard and a couple of meetings I was late for because I dared not exit the comfort room mid-telephone conversation. Who knows what they would have assumed I was doing in there.

The repetitive nature of these Off Periods was almost impossible to cope with initially. It was difficult to beat something you knew that you could only defeat for a few hours. The onslaught just kept coming. The only way to survive was one battle or skirmish at a time.

I did my best to minimise any impact on my management responsibilities through fastidious scheduling. At the beginning, the Off Periods were entirely predictable. It was easy to schedule around them. As the symptoms progressed, and I relied more and more on Sinemet, this became more of a challenge.

In the moments after the Sinemet became effective, I frequently asked myself why I felt the urge to keep working. I could simply stay home and suffer in private. There was the obvious, the promise I had made to my boss and then there was my fear of atrophy. Without mental exercise the brain shrinks. At forty-nine, I didn't dare to spend the next thirty-odd years without a purpose. I am convinced that without a challenge, big or small, you shrink and ultimately you die. As they say in the movie *The Shawshank Redemption* – 'get busy living or get busy dying'. I chose living.

Not all meetings were under my scheduling control. We were still engaged with the Federal Communications Commission and the Department of Justice and had to accept any time the staffers offered for meetings. There was a real possibility that an important meeting would be scheduled during an Off Period. The specialist suggested that I place my trust in a drug which had been on the International Olympic Committee Banned Drugs List for decades; beta blockers slow down the heartbeat, which can be highly beneficial in events like shooting where you need to fire at the target between beats. Obviously, the longer the interval between two consecutive pulses of the heart, the longer the shooter has to make sure her aim is true.

Four months into my assignment we had assembled all the leadership team and a group of highly capable and competitive former allies. We augmented with a team from Deloitte who acted as our systems integrator. The group coalesced nicely under extraordinary stress. It was a constant strain to make sure the environment was enjoyable. We instituted flexible hours and doled out autonomy and utilised every fun-inducing event we could conceive of. My favourite was undoubtedly St Patrick's Day when we engaged a bagpiper to play while we toasted progress with a shot of Irish whiskey, all forty of us by then.

We had taken on even more than I had imagined. The business risk here was our ability to convert, and this heavily factored into the price ATNI had paid. The financial markets were betting that our transition efforts wouldn't succeed. Everything about this project screamed 'runaway'. The risk clearly outweighed the rewards for me. Much as I wanted to cancel the endeavour and actually run away, I couldn't. This was my canvas. It certainly wasn't the perfect canvas, but it certainly was my last and only. So I decided to grab the opportunity with both hands.

* * *

In my earlier life, I had an experience quite similar to my time as CEO, in terms of venturing into the unknown to create an opportunity. Marcus O'Sullivan and I were two of the best young runners in Ireland at that time. Marcus was runner-up in the 1984 National Collegiate Athletic Association (NCAA) 1,500 metres and I was the 1983 champion. We struggled to get into international meets and were desperate to show that we belonged. There was no Google to search for an athletics meet's information and no email to contact the meet director.

Athletics was run by the International Amateur Athletics Federation (IAAF), and each member nation had an affiliate. In Ireland, the affiliate was called Bord Lúthchleas na hÉireann (BLE). To compete in an overseas meet, the International Secretary of BLE would contact a counterpart in the other country to arrange an invitation for an athlete to compete, then issue a permit for that meeting.

Our International Secretary arranged for Marcus O'Sullivan and me to compete in DN Galen Meet in Stockholm. A deal was struck that BLE would pay for our travel to Sweden. We would be reimbursed by the Swedish meet director, who would provide accommodation in the meet hotel. Our specific instructions were to queue up with the other athletes after the meet to collect the agreed-upon amount. Interestingly, we were only provided with one-way tickets, and were instructed to ask the meet director to pay for the return trip.

We arrived in Stockholm and made our way to the hotel. The lobby was a hive of activity. There were the spirited faces of well-known US sprinters and the sterner countenances of the eastern bloc athletes. All of this was a little intimidating for two young Irishmen. We immediately decided to get our room key and hide out until race time.

In those days, athletes were paid an appearance fee, which technically was contrary to the amateur rules of the sport. To prevent discovery, you were paid in cash by the promoter. First you had to queue outside his suite to collect what had been agreed, minus any arbitrary deduction he unilaterally decided to impose. Facing the wrath of an ill-tempered promoter could be quite intimidating; nobody looked forward to the ordeal.

The next day we raced over 1,500 m and finished second and third behind an American, Chuck Aragon. That relieved some of the angst of facing the meet director, but we still had to go through the process. We had to get him to pay for our way home. The line was long, but the meet director felt good about our performances and was happy to reimburse BLE for our one-way tickets. We informed him that BLE had not booked a return flight. The director empathised, but was adamant that a deal was a deal. Perhaps if there was a surplus at the end of the night, he would pay for a return ticket.

We had run well, but we needed more races to prepare for the Los Angeles Olympic Games later that summer. We decided to go to the post-meet party as a kind of reconnaissance move, see what plans the others had. We were improvising. Meetings in Europe did not complete until late in the evening. That combined with the bright Scandinavian nights and the residual adrenaline in our systems meant sleep was not on the cards. We met a very amicable Swede by the name of Kent Andersen. He was on the organising committee and one of the great characters on the circuits. We told him about our concerns and that we were presently marooned in Stockholm.

He said, 'No, no, you're thinking about this all wrong. Many of the athletes here are going to a meet in Larvik in the morning. You both need to go and race there.'

We were all in. He said, 'Leave it to me, I will arrange everything. Just be at the bus at nine in the morning.'

It was well after 2am when Kent advised us to join the group to Norway. Seven hours to the bus departure. Kent must have had a rough night because he couldn't be roused the next morning for love nor money. Now we were in a difficult spot. Our benefactor was a no-show and apparently had told nobody about his commitment. We weren't even sure that he had the authority to speak for the Norwegians. This was a critical moment. The meet director hadn't come through with the return fare. We had to get home from somewhere – it may as well be Norway as Sweden.

We decided to stow away on the Larvik bus. Athletes were simply getting on. Nobody was checking a roster. We got on and took a seat at the back. I think we had Sony Walkmans or some other prehistoric analogue music player. We put on a tape and lowered our heads and kept them down. An official boarded the bus and did a headcount. Luckily, he didn't appear to reconcile the count with any prescribed forecast. He did note the headcount in a little notebook as he passed us, thirty-one. Suddenly, the coach lurched forward, and we were on our way. We rode along acting like we belonged, nervous as you can imagine. As we neared the airport that same official gave out instructions that they would assemble in the group check-in area. Everyone piled off the bus, gathered their bags and waited as the official spoke with the agent. We were sure our cover was blown. We weren't on any list. Our hearts raced as we observed the discourse. Then he flipped open the book he had written in, and I was sure he said 'thirty-one'. The agent began counting boarding passes. I tried to keep track of her count, but the last number I heard was twenty-eight. The official took the boarding passes and spun round to face us. We were petrified with fear as he spoke to the group.

'Follow me to the gate. I have the passes,' he said.

Maybe, just maybe, we could be safe. Sure enough, we got to the gate, and he handed a boarding pass to each athlete as we walked by him to enter the departure lounge area, including athletes numbers thirty and thirty-one. He wished us a safe flight and then he left. We had survived, but we still faced risk. Would the Larvik meet director let us run and how would we get home?

We loitered around the edges of the group until boarding and picked up some intelligence from group members. Apparently, many were destined for the Bislett Games in Oslo, three days after the meeting in Larvik.

Stakes were just raised. Perhaps we could parlay good runs in Larvik into an opportunity to race at the iconic stadium that had seen so many world records. We were part of the tally now, and it would have disrupted all the logistics if suddenly the numbers were down by two. It should be plain sailing until we got to the hotel in Larvik. We disembarked the aircraft like two undercover agents who had infiltrated a gang and boarded a coach for the three-hour trip to Larvik. There, we found ourselves in another queue in the meeting hotel. The back of the queue to be exact. If there was to be a brouhaha, we'd rather not embarrass ourselves in front of fellow competitors.

Finally, it was our turn. We decided to throw ourselves at the mercy of the director. We explained our predicament, told him about our new friend Kent and how he had encouraged us to come to Larvik.

'Are you any good?' muttered the director.

Fortunately, we had placed well in Stockholm, but still he was uncertain. I was bothered until Marcus reached into his backpack and pulled out a copy of the June edition of *Track & Field News* which contained year to date standings. To my relief we both featured in those rankings. Almost convinced, he nonetheless instructed us to sit in the corner and wait. Then, Kent Andersen breezed in with a second group of athletes. We rushed at him and pleaded that he intercede. Turns out Kent was happy to oblige, and he was equally persuasive.

Marcus ran well and won, and I managed to finish fourth, a little more than a second behind.

Marcus turned the tables on the American who had beaten us both earlier in the week. Sven Arne Hansen, the meet director for the renowned Bislett Games, was in attendance and saw Marcus's fine win. He duly invited Marcus to run in the Dream Mile a few days later. Marcus being the great friend that he is insisted that I be invited also. Sven agreed, and more importantly he agreed to pay for our travel home. I managed to win the 3,000m in that marvellous stadium and take some good scalps to burnish my reputation over the 3,000m distance. Marcus performed well in the Dream Mile, and we were rewarded with a little cash.

All's well that ends well. We were prepared to accept the consequences of our decision to stow away to Larvik because the benefit easily outweighed that risk. An introduction to the professional athletics community was paramount to our emerging careers. Being stranded in Norway was not much different to being stranded in Sweden. At worst we could throw ourselves at the mercy of the Irish embassy in Oslo. At the end of the day, we discounted the risk and prioritised the upside.

\* \* \*

I once heard someone say that your happiness is directly proportional to your acceptance and inversely proportional to your expectations. A simple enough concept, but hard to execute. I struggled mightily with both. It is difficult to rationalise downgrading your software to an earlier, less ambitious version. I was wired to set goals and the conquest of those goals fed my self-worth. The target had been world championships or Olympic teams and now it was getting dressed. I was part capable and part incapable, which was torture. Some days I was ready to take on the biggest challenges, other days not so much.

The acknowledgement that I needed breaks throughout the day was my first concession. I lowered expectations regarding my work effort and relied on the team we were building to do the heavy lifting. As expected, the team was immensely capable. Other than the occasional call centre or store visit, travel was minimal. I travelled occasionally to DC to fulfil my role as a member of the executive committee of the wireless trade association.

The combination of Lewis Langston's persistence, the steady hands of Brian Taylor, Lesa Handly, Dan Deem and CJ Duvall and their teams along with the remarkable Deloitte as systems integrator made the systems conversion a success. We performed the conversion in two stages. The second phase two months later covered ten times as many customers. We learned from the first and fixed all the major bugs identified in that phase before the second undertaking.

After a couple of years running the business, it became evident that we were swimming in the deep end of the pool. We were the ninth largest wireless operator in the US, but we were over a hundred times smaller than the top two. To offer nationwide coverage we needed to roam on the larger carrier's networks which wasn't affordable. Plus, there were 4G network upgrades required and 5G looming on the horizon. Spectrum and capital would be essential for both which would be a real challenge for us.

We knew that AT&T coveted our spectrum because of its ideal bandwidth and how nicely it complimented their holdings. They showed interest, and we began to negotiate the terms of a sale with them. These discussions can be lengthy and often amount to nothing, but around November we seemed to gain traction. It was imperative that negotiations didn't become public before a deal was announced.

As November drifted into December, two hugely important events were about to clash. A possible deal announcement date and my annual Christmas trip to Ireland to see my eighty-six-year-old mother. Patty and the boys visited my homeland every summer, but the Christmas visit was just my mother and me. She relished our time together. I delayed my departure a week and then another week to allow the slipping announcement date to grip. Finally, there were no further weeks to rearrange, and I had to cancel my trip. I promised I would return home in the new year, and we would have more time and perhaps visit the family homestead. I could hear the disappointment in my mother's voice when I told her. She didn't fully understand the significance of the conflicting event or why it all had to be so confidential, but like all devoted mothers, she accepted the disappointing turn of events.

The deal date slipped to the new year, further jeopardising my plans to make a flying visit. Then real life took over. I received a call from my sister telling me Mom was in hospital. Out of the blue, she was admitted the previous day. My sister advised me to come home promptly. I was terribly annoyed that the continual delays had needlessly cancelled my annual mother-son time. I assembled the team, explained the situation and made sure everyone knew their assignments. Thankfully they all understood and were prepared to cover for me.

I caught a flight home to Ireland the next afternoon and was at my mother's bedside the following morning. Thankfully, she was alert, but not vibrant. She could speak, but not conversationally; she was interested, but not engaged. She was nonetheless glad to see me. My siblings allowed us time to catch up. Mom wanted to know what was happening at work. She had run the family business for years after my father died, and she fully understood capital investment and cash flow constraints.

After she listened to my tale of how I sorry I was to have put work first, I told her I loved her and she responded in remarkable fashion, 'I love all of you equally'.

Extraordinary, no favourites to the bitter end, but also some reticence about repeating the words, 'I love you.' Many of my mother's generation had an aversion to such open expressions of affection. It was just understood that you loved your children. I remember after 9/11, when many of us realised that we shouldn't take the joys of life for granted nor the people we loved most, I told my mother that I loved her for the first time as an adult. Like I said, the Irish are frugal with the use of 'I love you.' She thought for a few seconds and responded with a classic.

'Francis, you know, we all love you too.'

I've thought about that not so casual response since and made these observations. She always called me Francis when she wanted my attention. She had my full attention. The 'you know' was her way of saying, 'why are you bringing up the obvious? and the use of 'we' indicated that she was uncomfortable with 'I love you'. So, she dragged my siblings into it. I had continued to remind her of my affection over the ensuing years, and I believed she had grown accustomed to it.

My mother had been admitted to the hospital with suspected pneumonia, something that can be easily cured. But three days into her hospitalisation, something was clearly awry. The previous day, doctors felt her heart was not strong enough to fight off the infection. A scan of her heart was required, and because the hospital did not have the appropriate scanning equipment, she had been taken by taxi across town to another hospital. She was in her pyjamas and dressing gown with her winter coat over them. The day before I arrived, she was transferred to the bigger hospital for continuing treatment.

She was in the same unit that my father had been in when he died. I never saw his hospital bed, because I was too young, but I did see my mother's. The ward was essentially a double-wide corridor. Patients were being moved to a brand-new ward that very day, and there were orderlies and porters in our hair the whole time. Power tools were brandished as they detached fixtures for the move and dismantled beds for transfer. They were callously working around my mother. When we complained about the circumstances, she was given a semi-private room. Although she had supplemental insurance, there were no private rooms to be had.

A dying eighty-six-year-old woman with her family around her was forced to share her final moments. We had very little privacy – we were only separated from the patient in the next bed by a thin curtain. We could hear the other patient speaking on her phone, oblivious to a precious life leaving this world feet away.

It reminded me of the Oscar Wilde quote which I have modified to suit the occasion: 'To lose one parent may be regarded as a misfortune; to lose both *in the same place* looks like carelessness'. I added 'in the same place'. Carelessness at the very least.

I have many misgivings and not providing more honour in her final hours still gnaws at me. In fairness, it all happened so quickly. The attending doctor met with my siblings and me to give us his prognosis. The scan revealed cancer on her heart.

'Can it be treated?' one of my sisters asked.

'No, because of where it is and her age.'

'How long does she have?' one of us asked.

'Not long,' was his reply.

I asked, 'Months?' to which he shook his head.

He shook similarly when I followed with weeks and nodded when I said days, adding, 'She could go fast.'

The end came quickly for my mother. She died peacefully three days later, four days after I arrived in town. Thank God my sister had the foresight to alert me to the danger. Thank God I had a team who were prepared to cover for me.

Patty and our boys dropped everything and travelled to Ireland four days later. We laid my mother out in the drawing room of her home until the funeral, an old country tradition that my boys did not understand, especially since we were staying in my mother's house too. We all grew up that weekend.

The day after the funeral, we were on our way back to Arkansas, the boys to schoolwork and me to announce to our staff that they had a new employer. While I was preoccupied in Ireland, AT&T agreed in principle to buy AWCC. The agreement was signed a few hours after my return, and the press release prepared for circulation when the markets opened that morning.

We held an all-employee meeting immediately after the announcement. These announcements can be awkward affairs. On the one hand, the team needs to remain focused and diligent in case the deal fails the regulatory approval hurdle, and the pieces of the business have to be picked up. On the other hand, the team is rightfully worried about their job prospects. Hopefully, you have negotiated severance conditions and assurances that your employees will be given opportunities in the bigger enterprise.

The entire experience, being by my ailing mother's side while simultaneously monitoring my phone for updates on deal progress, was discomforting at best. When you add in the physical and mental compromises caused by Parkinson's, you get a dastardly scenario that you hope never repeats.

Losing my mother under those conditions caused me to reevaluate. I was at a crossroads anyway. I was first out the door at AT&T, and likely my business career was over. In the first few months after the close of the AT&T deal, I received head-hunter calls for a few desirable roles; I feared I had lost the capacity to lead and perhaps even contribute. Disability was hurtling toward me like a runaway train.

The hits kept coming. Three weeks after my mother's passing, Patty's father died. In the end, his death was unexpected as he was doing well. His condition forced him to undergo a surgical procedure which he did not survive. Turns out we made a wise choice in deciding not to leave

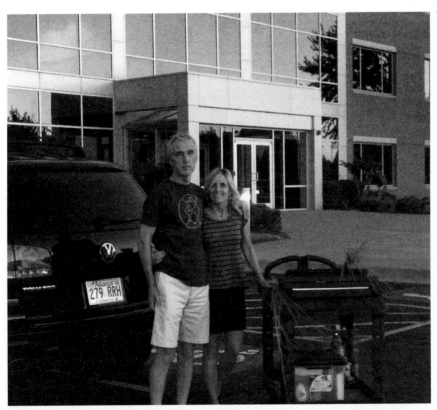

20 September 2013. The last day at Alltel after the acquisition by AT&T.

Little Rock. Apart from missing that week with my mother, we wisely prioritised family over business. The sale of AWCC essentially marked the end of my career. I had the opportunity to reset expectations and to work on acceptance.

My kids were growing up in front of me, I had lost loved ones, and a business challenge almost buried me. I was truly serving a life sentence. Parkinson's had eroded my abilities as a parent, husband and manager. But I had made it. I bent, but didn't break.

## CHAPTER 7

# BLOCK OUT DISTRACTIONS

After the AT&T buyout, I rejoined my former colleagues in the consulting business, but in truth I wasn't much use to them. I still received calls about work opportunities; but eventually word got out that I had Parkinson's.

Adjusting expectations was imperative. I had to calibrate my effort to a level I was capable of attaining. The trick was to manage any adjustment so that there remains something to reach for. Clearly, I was in a disarmament phase. Like the military after a conflict, I was drawing down weapons, shelving armoured vehicles and cancelling future weapons spending. I was in reverse gear. Each day I lost a little more of certain skills or the ability to perform a particular task. People always say you never forget how to ride a bike. My experience has been different. When you haven't ridden for a while and you have compromised balance, riding a bike is not going to happen no matter how deep you dig into the memory bank. The very fact that I have lowered the bar to accommodate an ailing body still rankles.

Perhaps I am doomed to lose more essential skills, but are there new skills I can acquire to replace them? Offset the losses?

I am a firm believer in neuroplasticity and have no doubt that acquiring new talents or enjoying different experiences creates new pathways in the brain. I could try to master a language, listen to music, learn an instrument. Visiting new places and making new friends are other alternatives. Accomplishments are a step forward not another step in an aimless retreat. It is a small sign of new growth.

I struggled too with acceptance. For many years, my first thought every morning was, 'Am I better?' There is a moment as you greet each day, half a moment really, right before cognition fully kicks in, where everything is a blank canvas waiting for you to don that day's perspective. In that instant, I could enjoy the illusion that I had made an overnight recovery. Similarly, if I have a good day where I can walk and talk. I experience that sensation. Those moments overwhelm me emotionally. The thought of being cured is that powerful. It may sound pitiful, but I was holding out hope that maybe the whole deal was a bad dream. Then the cramping would kick in and jolt me back to reality.

At my mother's funeral, I greeted an acquaintance whose father had been diagnosed with Parkinson's. She relayed that he no longer had Parkinson's, but with all the people in line to offer condolences it wasn't the time to provide details. I asked her to email me a more complete update on what happened. I got the mail about a week later and attached was an article from a British newspaper about a man whose Parkinson's turned out to be Lyme disease. It seems not to be so rare an occurrence. Her father had that exact experience. A neurologist diagnosed Parkinson's, and he took Sinemet to treat his tremor. Somehow, he learned of tick-borne diseases, and a doctor prescribed six weeks of antibiotic treatment, which killed the infection and rid him of his tremor.

Now, this wasn't an urban legend. This was a neighbour whose house I had been in as a kid, whose daughter went to school with my twin sisters.

A cure for him could surely work for me too. I had to know more so I arranged to call him. It was all true. He had been bitten by a sheep tick while fishing in Galway. When a tremor appeared, Parkinson's was an easy diagnosis. Once he was alerted to outbreaks of Lyme disease being carried by sheep ticks, he remembered the bite and put two and two together. After a course of Doxycycline, an antibiotic, the Parkinson's symptoms simply vanished.

In the majority of cases, it takes just four to six weeks of Doxycycline to clear the body of the toxins. Lyme can also be chronic and debilitating. I had been bitten by ticks on numerous occasions and was well aware of the challenge of removing the tick with the head intact. The head burrows into your flesh and generally remains *in situ* no matter what extraction technique is deployed. I recall on one occasion a friend suggested that I douse the annoying creature in mayonnaise to smother it and force it to release its death grip. This apparent sage advice turned out to be a lark, but it worked.

A key element of a Lyme diagnosis is the role of stress. The disease can lie dormant for many years after the offending bite and make its appearance after a stressful event in your life. I could check that box as well. The stress of losing a dream job could easily have precipitated the sudden onset of PD-like symptoms. The first symptom appeared the day after the purchase by Verizon was completed. The story lined up nicely; all boxes checked. I now needed to find a doctor to treat me. It turns out Lyme disease is quite controversial. Indeed, many in the medical community deny its existence, or at least the existence of the chronic variety. I was fortunate to find a local doctor who was familiar with the disease. He performed a battery of blood tests, confirming that I indeed had the disease. However, it was my medical history, mainly the stress-induced onset, that was convincing.

The approved six weeks of Doxycycline didn't work any particular magic. I still had Parkinson's symptoms. It seemed logical to conclude that I had the chronic version. All the evidence supported that view. I found an out-of-state expert in chronic Lyme's treatment and arranged an appointment. This specialist came with a reputation. He believed that a rigorous and prolonged regime was sometimes necessary to combat the more stubborn chronic variety. The standard insurance guidelines approved four to six weeks of antibiotics, so the only option was for the patient to pay. Judging by the number of people in the waiting room, there were plenty of volunteers.

The walls in his offices were covered in framed, handwritten letters of appreciation and gratitude from people whose lives he had improved. There were books and magazines strewn on every horizontal surface mentioning his commitment to the cause. I anxiously awaited his entry. Anyone who inspires a catalogue of sterling reviews should be able to help. What would my saviour look like? Would he agree with my doctor's diagnosis?

Parkinson's had a firm grip on my body at this point. Off Periods had become Off Mornings or Off Afternoons. I experienced full body shaking for four to six hours a day. Uncontrollable shaking that even the most ardent deep breathing could not assuage. While I waited for the doctor that morning, I had one of these 'seizures' in the waiting room. An orderly was walking by and saw the commotion. He immediately grabbed me in a tight clinching hug and waited for the shaking to abate. No amount of hugging was going to solve this issue and he released me into my own care. Unfortunately, the doctor did not witness this event, but he heard all about it.

I was also struggling with foggy headedness. My brain was shrouded in dense pea soup. It hurt to think, to process, to keep up in a conversation. I couldn't make decisions, small or large. I had no interest and no energy. I was a mess. I had just been introduced to cramping. Thankfully, the cramps were confined to my feet. Every morning, my big toe would curl under, and no amount of force could loosen Parkinson's vice-like grip.

The doctor arrived, curious to meet the patient who had the seizure-like event. He had a commanding presence, and his manner was on the belli-cose side. He seemed especially busy or at least gave the impression that he was. He introduced me to his Physician's Assistant, one of four, and announced that she would take the primary role in my care, naturally over-seen by him. He was obviously super busy.

I ignored my better instincts. 'Yes, Doctor, I understand.'

He listened to my health history and read the test results I presented. He came to the expected and inevitable conclusion. 'You have Lyme Borreliosis Complex.'

What a relief. Finally, a get-out-of-jail card.

The doctor devised a cocktail of various antibiotics and provided a detailed typewritten protocol to abide by. He predicted significant improve-ment in three to four months, but forewarned that chronic Lyme can be difficult to shake off.

The protocol called for Omnicef 300mg, Azithromycin 500mg, and Mepron 750mg. Each was taken twice daily Monday, Wednesday and Friday. On Thursday and Friday, Flagyl 500mg was added twice daily. I was instructed to continue this scheme for two weeks followed by a week off and repeat for three to four cycles. The doctor had concluded that the full body shaking I was experiencing was neuropathic in nature and proscribed the anti-convulsants Neurontin and Lamictal.

I felt properly encouraged as I checked out. The nurse had a stack of pill containers waiting for me at the counter. I knew that insurance would not cover any antibiotic treatment beyond the initial six weeks, but I had expected to receive a script to present at my local pharmacy. Turns out the doctor's office was selling the antibiotics. Although I was surprised, I was happy to pay for them on the spot. Travelling home with all these drugs made the journey a little more exciting. I was crossing state lines too, which raised trepidation levels further.

Flying home with Patty I could barely contain my excitement. I was ready to begin the regime. I told her my first step was to inform my neurologist of my good fortune. I planned on thanking him and notifying him that I would not need his care in the foreseeable future. If I believe in something, I am all in. I believe in the power of positivity and have long quoted the words attributed to Henry Ford, 'If you think you can or you think you can't, you're right'. No half measures then. If I really believed, I had to act like it. I had to cut all the lifeboats loose. I thanked my neurologist and placed all my energy into combating a tick.

Put your heart into the enterprise. This characteristic became both an advantage and a hindrance. I allowed my tenacity to dominate and, ultimately, to cloud my judgement. Over the next couple of years, I doubled down on my resolve. Such was my conviction that I would beat my diagnosis.

In many ways my adherence to this mad convention reminded me of the lead-up to the 1988 Olympic Games. At the time, Ireland had a cornucopia of talented middle-distance runners; we had eight milers who had run 3:55 or faster for a mile. A team of four Irish milers from that group still holds the World 4 x 1 mile relay record thirty-seven years later. I have the privilege of being one of the four, along with Marcus, Ray Flynn and

Eamonn Coghlan.

Irish milers were in demand on the international athletics circuit, and there was money to be made in appearance fees – fees paid to high-level athletes to run a particular race. Track and Field was a sport in transition. It was on a journey to discard its amateur past and embrace a professional future. Not everyone agreed with this seismic shift.

The International Amateur Athletic Federations (IAAF) had created an artificial but artful step designed ostensibly to protect the athletes' amateur status. This was merely a charade because the IAAF solely determined amateur status and could have just as easily decided to allow any athlete registered to be considered amateur. The IAAF passed a resolution that created a trust fund structure into which athletes' earnings were to be directed. This fund was to be administered by that country's national governing body, who then could retain a percentage for the inconvenience of managing those funds.

In 1987, the Irish national governing body, (BLE), formed a Trust Fund Committee, who then established trust accounts. That was their price of entry. Once trusts were operational, tariff collecting could begin. BLE estimated how much we had earned since enactment of the rule and applied the mandated percentage. We offered $10,000 to settle. Our offer was refused, and there was no counter-offer.

At a meeting in Seville, two senior officials offered a twenty per cent reduction on the previous demand. We refused and our refusal was relayed to the annual congress of BLE representatives held in Castlebar, County Mayo that December. This sparked outrage among the attendees, who called for heads to roll.

One delegate, Fr John O'Donnell, a former president of BLE, was quoted as saying, 'If we have to lose three or four international athletes, so be it.' Nice to know we could be dispensed with so incontrovertibly.

Participation in the following year's Olympics was in jeopardy. There were numerous skirmishes throughout the spring of 1988, mostly in print. BLE told the press on many occasions that we would not be selected for the Seoul Olympics. We never doubted that BLE were serious, but it was still alarming to see the threat in writing.

I received a letter dated 10 May 1988 that said, 'Please remember that any violation or non-compliance with these rules and regulations will result in INSTANT EXCLUSION FROM IRISH INTERNATIONAL PANELS AND TEAMS AND A LIFETIME AND WORLDWIDE BAN FROM ALL COMPETITIONS.' Suddenly, the situation had gone nuclear. Ben Johnson would only get a four-year ban for anabolic steroids in the 100m in Seoul, but we deserved a lifetime ban for keeping what we had fairly earned.

The five of us subject to such an extraordinary censure were principled and not prepared to be bullied. BLE had a new rule on their side. Everyone knew the rule was a stopgap measure until the inevitable – full-on professionalism. What we encountered were the last twitches of a dying system.

The whole country read about the saga almost weekly in the newspapers. This was no way to prepare for the Olympic Games. We were certain we would be banned. I'm not suggesting for a minute we were at the vanguard of a movement, but we did feel the issue was bigger than just the five of us.

Only the intervention of a wealthy businessman from Dundalk, Neil McCann, suspended hostilities. Mr McCann loved athletics and couldn't stand all the bickering and resentment. He placed the exact amount in dispute in escrow until after the games, at which time the parties would meet

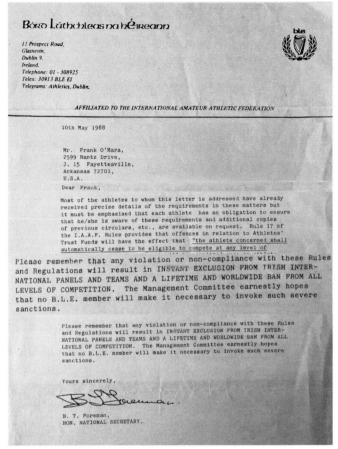

**10 May 1988. The letter sent by the Irish athletics body three months before the Olympics.**

and settle the dispute without the pressures of the games. This arrangement allowed us to compete in Seoul. Mind you, after all the anxiety of the previous months and inconsistent preparation, our performances were not what we hoped for. Though to be fair to Marcus O'Sullivan and John Doherty, they both made the finals.

Both sides were a little chastened when we arrived home after the games. Nobody was interested in our little drama. BLE had lost their biggest leverage, Olympic Games participation, and we had not distinguished ourselves on the track. BLE were eager to close out the tawdry affair and they negotiated with our agent, Kim McDonald, a settlement that put us all out of our misery. The terms mandated that we pay a one-time penalty, place all our future earnings in a trust and allow BLE to withhold a percentage.

The embers of professionalism were stoked by other athletes in other countries. The first big step toward abolition of trust funds was late in 1992 when the British Athletics Federation cancelled its trust fund levy. A full year after this event, BLE were still bellied up at the trough. The IAAF rule concerning trust funds was still in place, and they were simply enforcing the rules. They were like a captain going down with his ship. And yes, that ship was about to sink.

We took matters into our hands and wrote BLE a letter dated 20 December 1993, in which we said, 'In view of these changes over the last twelve months, it seems wholly inappropriate that we should continue to pay a levy to BLE.'

So, I had plenty of experience with naysayers. There were many sceptics on the topic of Lyme disease, particularly Chronic Lyme, my stated version. The ingrained opposition is best evidenced by an encounter I had with a former colleague who happens to be the spouse of a doctor. One day, while I was gardening in our front yard, she walked by and asked how I was doing. I told her about my Parkinson's escape plan. I could see the disapproval on her face as she declared that it would never work.

Our willingness to stand up to the Irish athletics federation was a source of encouragement and provided sustenance for my adherence to the treatment plan. I had chosen my direction and charged headlong into my treatment. The antibiotic regime is referred to as 'pulsing'. You pound the patient with antibiotics four or five days a week for three weeks followed by a week's respite, and you repeat. Because Lyme is so nefarious it can adapt to any protocol. Accordingly, the regime has to be constantly changed to confuse it. In total I tried over ten different antibiotics in both oral and IV forms. The doctor varied the cycles endlessly, two weeks off, three off, four on, three on. Who knew a tick could be so ingenious. New antiseizure medicines were also introduced to combat the shaking.

All these antibiotics were likely to play havoc with my gastrointestinal system; accordingly I was advised to perform a number of purification techniques. I was told to adopt a gluten-free diet, which Patty had to endure. Copious amounts of probiotics were also on the menu. We became familiar with kimchi and kombucha. Finally, there were saunas to sweat out the toxins created by the clash between the antibiotics and the invader.

## CHAPTER 8

# STICK WITH IT

I noticed a trend immediately. On the weeks I was on antibiotics, I began to experience full-body shaking; a constant shuddering similar to the sensation you felt starting a car with the choke fully extended in the seventies. The engine revving and the car vibrating. During the on weeks, this shaking totalled four to six hours a day. Conversely, there was a noticeable decrease in tremors in the week off antibiotics. I was assured this was all part of the 'kill-off' process, and I simply had to tough it out.

The Lyme doctor ordered a Dat-Scan, which is essentially brain imaging taken after administration of a radioactive pharmaceutical, a marker that allows a technician to see changes in the size of the compromised region of the brain. My result showed a decrease on both sides, but more substantial on the right side. Interestingly, the right side of the brain controls the left side of the body. The first and worst symptoms I experienced were on my left side. The technician's opinion was Parkinson's. The Dat-Scan result was a red flag. When I quizzed the doctor about this anomaly, he claimed the result supported his contention that I suffered from Parkinson's-Presenting Lyme disease. I should have demonstrated scepticism, but instead discarded all common sense. I went along with him, happily knowing I was on the right track. The cost of entry into this club of believers was the suspension of neurological treatment. I missed the periodic adjustments to medication that may have ameliorated some of the disease progression. I could have supplemented my current treatment with agonists that accentuate Levodopa's efficacy and coping strategies like diet and exercise.

Along with the increased shaking, cramping had become a reliable foe. What had begun in my feet over a few months moved into my calves. The sensation was deep in the muscle tissue without necessarily being observable on the exterior. These cramps could not be released by manipulation. It felt like I was being attacked from within.

A few months later again, the cramping made an assault on my neck, forcing my head to tilt downward from the severity of the contraction. If it wasn't a long attack, often other facial muscles would get involved, most often the muscles that control the eyelids. These neck cramps were to be a constant fixture in my life. They would eventually require drastic action to remedy.

My resolve was definitely tested as my condition deteriorated. There was little to show after months of oral antibiotics. I was downtrodden, but with the encouragement of the doctor I was determined to stay the course. He kept repeating that this was *never* going to be easy. I have always believed there is merit to hanging around the hoop; eventually you get a rebound.

I was reminded on every visit not to be disheartened, that good things come to those who follow the prescribed protocol. I drew on the rough start to my college athletics career whenever I felt doubt. My disappointing start and eventual success were an early introduction to 'sticking with it'.

It seemed the more I yearned for success, the more success managed to evade me. There is a point in your struggle when the effort required can seem overwhelming. The more you struggle in races, the harder you work in training. Working hard fruitlessly only raises frustration levels. You are so consumed with doubt, you can't seem to improve. You push too hard when you just need to let it come to you, a bit like a striker in football who is on a cold streak. You watch others perform with more than a little envy.

Too often, I have sat on the sidelines because of injury watching others achieve what I aspired to. More than a little jealousy can set in if you're not careful. I truly believe that you have arrived as a fully mature adult when you can embrace success of a teammate or work companion or friend.

Oscar Wilde summed it up nicely when he said, 'Anybody can sympathise with the sufferings of a friend, but it requires a very fine nature to sympathise with a friend's success.'

My Lyme treatment forced me to draw on all my resources. I reminded myself that I had been in some dark places in a previous life, had faced doubt about my ability to cope, but had persevered. A dreadful performance in the 1988 Olympics springs to mind, a shameful run that still annoys. I survived that embarrassment. Surely, I could do the same fighting this tick.

My Lyme disease doctor reiterated that the increase in symptoms was all part of the kill-off process. He even put a name to this kill-off; he referred to it as a Herxheimer Reaction. This term describes a short-term detoxification reaction to certain antibiotic treatments. The kill-off results in an inflammatory response causing multiple symptoms. It is not uncommon to experience a flu-like reaction including headache, joint and muscle pain, body aches, general malaise, sweating, chills, nausea or brain fog.

He advised that I take lots of Epsom salt baths and drink litres of water. The very fact that I was experiencing many of these symptoms was evidence that toxins were being released in my body, and therefore the antibiotics were in mortal combat with the dreaded tick infection.

Regardless of whatever misgivings she may have had, Patty continued to support my madness. She drove me to my many detox sessions at a local sauna or therapist. She never wavered. Mind you, she did raise an eyebrow when I began sessions at a chiropractic clinic that offered special detox foot baths. My kids seemed a little less convinced, but they didn't see me with the same frequency and likely could see the deterioration more clearly.

At the pinnacle of this phase of my treatment, I had an oddly reinforcing experience. Suzanne Woody, my massage therapist, who I began to see as my initial response to the earlier running problem, had learned various new techniques that may help her treat me as part of her required continuing education. One of those skills was Craniosacral Therapy, an alternative therapy where the practitioner regulates the cerebral spinal fluid to remove any interruptions in the flow. Previous events can create emotional responses that become trapped in our bodies and disrupt the flow. Emotions have a powerful effect on our psyches as well as our bodies. Within Craniosacral Therapy, there is a process designed to expunge these feelings. This process is called SomatoEmotional Release (SER).

During one of our sessions, I experienced one of these emotional responses. In fairness, it had been a particularly arduous week of pulsing antibiotics, but nonetheless, the response happened. I must have fallen asleep on the table; Suzanne swears she doesn't have any hypnotic talents. I found myself in either a trance or a light sleep, and I pictured a scene straight out of Monty Python. I was outside a medieval castle which was under attack from within. The attackers were the poisonous toxins that the tick had deposited into my body, the castle. As the fight raged on, the castle kept expelling dead organisms through holes at the base of the walls. In the aberration, I featured pushing a cart around the dried-up moat, picking up the dead organisms as they were ejected. I even gave the tick a name, Marvin.

I snapped out of it, a little startled but excited by the dream. I felt the psychological event reflected reality and established that I was on the correct path. This had to be the Herxheimer Effect in action. Suzanne immediately asked that I draw what I had seen. My depiction showed a castle with the shadow of a giant tick looming over it belching out spherical toxins from its mouth.

I don't know if that episode makes me look foolish, but it certainly confirms the power of the mind. So, I put my shoulder to the grindstone for the next push, the next round of kill-off. I was absolutely convinced that I had Marvin cornered.

Since we now had the incorrigible tick in our crosshairs, we needed to apply extra pressure. The doctor suggested I have a procedure at a hospital near his office to install a port in my chest. A port is placed in a vein in the chest close to the heart and provides for intravenous administration. We could pump it directly into the blood now and really pile the pressure on.

That night while at dinner with Patty and our son, Colin, we noticed that my shirt was turning red. We initially thought it was an untimely ketchup stain, but when the blemish continued to grow, we knew it was something much different. It turned out to be blood leaking from the surgery wound around the port. We left Colin to pay up and dashed off to the Emergency Room. When he arrived, we were still waiting as the blood stain continued to grow. Colin insisted that I stand in front of the triage nurse until I was seen. Just as well I did since the ER staff had to call in a member of the surgical team from earlier in the day to staunch the bleeding.

Patty was trained to operate the port, attach the IV bags and use a saline cleanse. So, for the next eight months, I sat around the house with an IV attached to my chest and made Netflix my best friend. Patty soldiered on too, always worrying that I would fall asleep and neglect to clip off the line when the bag ran out and allow air bubbles to enter my bloodstream. There were some scary moments. We had purchased a pole to hang the bags of fluid from. The principles of gravity apply so you must have a height differential between the port and the solution. Not surprisingly, if the heart is above the bag's level, blood will flow into the tube and ultimately … Well, you can imagine you need to avoid this scenario.

On one occasion, I needed to use the bathroom. I undid the bag from the pole and carried it with me. The liquid continued to drip as I shuffled along. We lived in an older home, and the downstairs bathroom was tiny, no bigger than that found on a train. Furthermore, it was under the stairs and had a sloped ceiling. Positioning yourself in the space was quite a feat. In the process of navigating the restricted confines, I lost track of the bag's elevation. Next time I checked on its welfare, I saw that half the tubing was now red. There was blood in the line, and it was travelling toward the bag and not at insignificant pace. I panicked and shouted out to Patty who immediately responded. She called the nurse who came weekly to change the dressing. To our relief she answered instantly; she knew we were amateurs. She instructed us to sit down and raise the bag as high as possible. Immediately, the blood began travelling in the opposite direction and eventually the line was clear again. It was a frightening experience for both of us.

We continued the pulsing protocol. The 'on' weeks were even more awful as the symptoms began to multiply in terms of both intensity and frequency and new symptoms made an appearance. I had difficulty with the simplest of tasks, talking and walking. Now we really had this tick cornered, he was angry and fighting back. We were close. At least, that was what I was repeatedly told.

My friends who were sceptical at the beginning clearly thought I had lost touch, and those who had believed had become sceptical. Everyone around me could see the deterioration. Even I had to admit the decision to pursue chronic Lyme treatment looked foolhardy. I was tired, dead tired; I had only gotten worse. It was time to give up on that hope and face my reality. I should have doubted the whole scheme much earlier than I did. The writing was on the wall long before I saw it.

My next visit to the Lyme doctor was the last. I told him I was done fighting ticks. Strangely, he suggested that I would need to begin a maintenance course of oral antibiotics. There was no end to his optimism. Well, there was to mine. He was still talking about 'kill-off' the last I heard. I do feel he had my best interests at heart, but he was too myopic to see we weren't making progress. Given that we don't know what causes Parkinson's disease, it is plausible that mine originated with a tick bite. However, the destruction of dopamine-producing cells could not be reversed, so whether I had Parkinson's or Parkinson's Presenting Lyme was really irrelevant.

I had the port removed the following month. My regret is I may have accelerated the regressive curve of my disease. At forty-eight years of age, I was considered early onset, and the general prognosis is a slow progression. Mine has been rapid, and that may be the price I had to pay for believing I could conquer this disease. Perhaps a little acceptance was in order.

I found out that there is no negotiation with Parkinson's. It has its own agenda, its own pace. It is going to win eventually. The only thing to be decided is when it can declare victory. That, I can have a say in. I have come to an agreement with my uncooperative brain that I will sustain it as long as I can. I will continue to explore ways to keep neurological paths open, I will always have events to look forward to, I will rest, I will exercise.

Negotiation is a skill I thought I had mastered until I met Eamonn Coghlan. He was a masterful negotiator and he declared once that there is nothing you won't do for a price. I asked him what exactly he meant, and he replied. If you really don't want to do an event, ask for something ridiculous. If they acquiesce, then you are getting very well paid; if they decline you won't be disappointed. It's a win/win since you didn't want to participate in the first place.

I was in college and had mountains of work, which were about to consume me. I received a call enquiring if I would compete in a road race in the UK. The caller was pretty keen to have me on the starting line. I really didn't want to miss more classes, plus I had just returned from racing in Europe. The caller asked how much it would take to persuade me to travel back. I remembered Eamonn's advice and adopted his tactic instantly. I threw out a number that was triple what I would typically get paid. There was no immediate response, so I must have gotten close to the nub, but I really had no desire to compete. So, I increased my ask hoping he would decline.

'I have one more request.'

'Go on then.'

'I want to be flown over on the Concorde,' I proposed.

Concorde was a commercial airliner that flew supersonic. It took just over two hours to traverse the Atlantic from New York to London. A Boeing 747 in comparison took over six hours.

The caller hesitated. 'I'll have to think about that. Give me a few hours and I'll call you back.'

I put down the phone, confident that I had made a request beyond his reach. I firmly expected I would not hear from him again. I went back to my constitutional law book and the case of Lochner v New York.

True to his word, the race director called me before the day was through. It was bad news – or was it good news?

I grabbed the phone and stretched the long chord around the corner. 'Hello, this is Frank.'

'I'm calling to say we have a deal,' he said. 'You are on Concorde from JFK next Thursday. You'll be back on Sunday as requested.'

I was crestfallen, but managed to enquire, 'What time do I leave Fayetteville?'

'Depart at 11:40. Your ticket is prepaid and will be at the airport for you.'

I had mixed feelings. I was getting very well paid, and travel would be easy, but I missed so many classes because of travel to indoor meets, how would I explain this to my professors, who were just about tired of all my absences.

On the appointed Thursday, I flew to JFK and waited excitedly to board. The Concorde looked sleek and fast with its nose strangely down as if inspecting the ground. It was dwarfed by the mammoth 747s lined up in various liveries. It turned out to be as small inside as it appeared from the outside. There were twenty-five rows of four seats separated by a narrow aisle. What Concorde lacked in size was more than compensated for by the impeccable service and sheer speed. We had barely finished eating and the wheels were out for landing.

I made my way to the event location and prepared for the next morning's race. I knew I was in for a dogfight from a number of fine UK athletes. Somehow, I managed to win, barely. That evening I travelled back to Heathrow to catch the next morning's flight.

The next day I approached the check-in counter perplexed. I suspected from the indistinctive flight number that something was awry. The flight to Heathrow from Kennedy had a simple short number like BA 004. The number on my itinerary was BA 1256. I explained to the agent that I was flying the Concorde to JFK. She giggled and gleefully told me I must be mistaken. A Concorde ticket was clearly beyond my means.

'I am supposed to be on the Concorde. I flew here on it two days ago. There must be a mistake,' I urged.

That rattled her a little and she committed to checking the system notes. After quickly navigating between a few screens, she responded. 'I can see you flew over on the Concorde, but the booking is economy on the return.'

I had been outsmarted. Not only would I not fly supersonic, but I was flying economy. He had only promised to fly me over. I hadn't asked about the return journey. I gave a rueful smile and thought, *Well done, Mr Race Director, you got me.*

My attempt to outsmart the race director went a bit like my attempt to reach an agreement with Parkinson's, to forestall its forward march. It may take longer than Parkinson's wishes, but it will prevail. That I don't deny. Therein lies the difficulty of fighting diseases like Parkinson's.

They cannot be defeated, but that doesn't rule out a few pluses on my side of the ledger. Victory must be construed in different terms. Victory could be as simple as having a good day or as dramatic as taking a trip overseas. Victory is a life well lived or a day enjoyed.

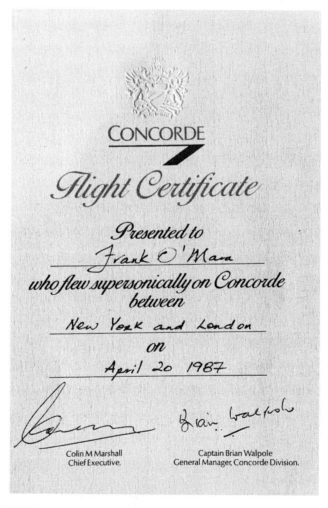

CONCORDE

*Flight Certificate*

*Presented to*

Frank O'Mara

*who flew supersonically on Concorde between*

New York and London

*on*

April 20 1987

Colin M Marshall
Chief Executive,

Captain Brian Walpole
General Manager, Concorde Division.

20 April 1987. A one-way journey on the Concorde.

## CHAPTER 9

# STAND FOR SOMETHING

One of the most formative experiences of my life occurred at an athletics meet. Without the internet and wi-fi, it was next to impossible for a young athlete to know a meet director's name, never mind their phone numbers. Everyone had a little address book with meet directors' contact information. Seasoned athletes were pestered for a glimpse into their enviable Rolodex.

These were the days before prize money when athletes were paid appearance fees. A reasonable appearance fee was merited if you had a title behind your name. That makes sense; a meet director has to put people in seats and sell the broadcast rights. How better to market a meet than the participation of multiple world champions or Olympic medallists?

There was one sure way to get on the starting line; the outside spot on the curve was reserved for pacemakers. Pacemakers – sometimes called 'rabbits' – are engaged to run a portion of the race at a quick pace to help other runners to a fast time. In return, there was an understanding that you would receive entry into partner meets and to that particular meet the following year. Plus, you were paid much better. I didn't have a bright, shiny title, so I struggled to get a spot in the big meetings.

The top tier of professional athletics was then called the Mobil Grand

Prix. I was asked to act as a pacemaker by Enrico Dionisi, the agent for Saïd Aouita, the Moroccan athlete who was dominant at 5,000m and vied with Steve Cram for the mantle of the world's number-one miler.

Enrico liked me and claimed this was a great opportunity for me. He said, 'If you can get Saïd to the three-quarter-mile mark in 2:48 in Zurich, I promise you race for yourself next.'

I was shocked at hearing 2:48, and I blurted my surprise. 'You can't be serious, 2:48?'

'Saïd is serious. You know he likes to go with a fast tempo.'

I was familiar with Saïd's application. He was as competitive as anybody I had ever seen. There were races he should have been beaten in that he simply refused to lose.

'When will I get to race myself?' I asked.

At which point he promised that I could race in Berlin two days later.

I didn't have a spot in either meet, so I had nothing to lose. And, if I could run 2:48, well, that would only be a harbinger of success for later races. A local Swiss athlete took the pace for the first two laps in 1:52, and then it was Saïd and me alone on the third lap. One hurting more than the other, but only one of us with a fourth lap remaining. Coming to the bell I could see the clock turn over from 2:48 to 2:49. As he passed me at the bell, I saw how much he was suffering and thought there was no way the world record would be broken tonight. He soldiered on and narrowly missed the world record with a final time of 3:46.9, amazing given how he had to drag himself round the track for an entire lap.

I then discovered that pace-making can be a trap. If you do the job too well, especially if you can get the race to the three-quarter-mile mark, then all the meets want you in that role. I was always a good judge of pace, and

I especially prided myself on gauging how the athlete behind was feeling. No point in running off and gapping the star. Better to keep him close and encourage him.

Enrico told me that Saïd had asked the meet director to arrange for me to act as a pacemaker two days later at the ISTAF Grand Prix meeting in Berlin.

'But you told me I could race for myself in Berlin.'

'I did, but you had to take him through in 2:48, and the pace was 2:49,' he responded.

'Okay, what do I get this time?'

'I will get you into the Brussels meeting. Just give it everything you got,' he urged.

It was a 1,500m on this occasion, three and three quarters laps of the track. I gave it my all and took him through in 2:48.4 for three laps. He was in similar pain as he swept by me with 280m left, but his huge capacity to turn himself inside out prevailed, and he broke his first world record. He was delighted and equally appreciative.

Enrico was true to his word, and I got a spot in the final Grand Prix of the season, The Van Damme Classic in Brussels. After my two pace-making assignments, I was primed to race well. I finished second to Spanish runner José Marie Abascal in a personal best time of 3:34.01.

My first major meet in Europe the following year was a mile in a stadium on the ocean in a warmer part of Europe. I was excited as Saïd Aouita was running the mile also and presumably the race would be quick. I knew I was in the best shape ever and ready to run fast. I was on good terms with Saïd and especially his agent, Enrico. The previous September, I had been invited to join Saïd's training group in Siena, Italy. I was very flattered to be considered, and I knew even at the time that it would have been a huge catalyst in my running career. I decided to reject the offer because of graduate school and a certain Patty Olberts with whom I had classes.

Declining the offer to train in Siena may have been the first sign that I didn't have the unbalanced nature that Sonia alluded to. If you believe that Siena was likely to have improved my performance, then I prioritised school and girlfriend higher. I have always believed in having choices and alternatives if something goes awry. I was building a bulwark to failure. In hindsight, it may appear I was not *all* in. This compromise of principles does not mean that I worked any less hard. Indeed, the following year, I upped my mileage significantly to prepare for the Olympic 5,000m in Seoul, Korea. After six weeks at training camp, I was so emaciated from overwork that Patty walked by me at the stadium. She did not recognise me; the shaved head didn't help. Just as well I was balanced after that performance. Or maybe it is the other way around. Either way, Ms O'Sullivan is correct. You need imbalance to be truly great.

Aouita wanted the mile world record he had barely missed in Zurich the prior year. I had ambitions of breaking the Irish record, which stood at 3:49.79. My best at that time was 3:52.30, so within reach. The afternoon of the meet, the starting line-ups were made available in the lobby. This was when I realised that Aouita *did* have plans to run fast – and those plans included me acting as his pacemaker again! As I read the starting line-ups, I noticed I had the designation 'P' alongside my name. 'P' for pacemaker.

It is generally not too difficult to spot someone with authority in a busy hotel lobby before a track meeting. They are the one with most athletes or agents hovering around them, staged purposefully to resolve the more mundane issues. The senior most meeting director was ensconced in a suite upstairs, leaving the operative in the lobby to manage the noise. After the heat sheets are delivered, there is no deficit of issues ranging from sprinters unhappy about lane draws to the departure time of the first bus.

I waited in orbit to relay my displeasure with the operative who was assigned first-level complaint resolution. I told him, 'Would you please tell the meet director that I don't want to pace-make?'

Then I realised I had not revealed the event or my name and quickly blurted out, 'O'Mara, mile, sorry.'

He flipped through a bundle of worn-looking sheets until he came to the mile field and revealed, rather flippantly, 'Saïd asked for you. He is going for the world record tomorrow.'

I replied that nobody had the courtesy to inform me, and I wouldn't have asked to race had I known this was a possibility.

He got the message and hurried off. This was an issue worthy of the meet director's ears. He wasn't gone long before he excitedly re-emerged with a message that the meet directors would pay what Berlin had paid me when Saïd broke the 1,500m record the previous year. That had indeed been my biggest payday; I was paid $5,000 to pace and a further $2,000 for the world record. In contrast, I was being paid $3,000 to race here. So I stood to make almost triple by running less.

It is easy to see how you can get sucked into pace-making. More money, less distance, but I wasn't in the sport for money. I had goals of my own. They were written in my training diary, a sure sign of my ambition. If you were brazen enough to commit to ink, you definitely meant business.

I bravely declared that I had a higher calling than making money and replied, 'I don't want to rabbit, please.'

His disbelief could not be hidden. His cheeks puffed up with rancour.

The mile was the cornerstone of the meeting, and a world record would cement the meet's reputation as one of the finest meets on the calendar.

Then a calm seemed to envelop him, as if he had figured out a solution. 'We will see what we can do about that,' he said and rushed off to the elevator. He had surmised that I was merely negotiating.

He returned and summoned me to follow him. 'The director wants you upstairs now,' he snarled. We rode up in the elevator together, not saying much, just counting the floors as they crawled by. We reached the top level and waited impatiently for the doors to open. In awkward situations like that, doors never open quickly, no matter how often you press the button or how loud the beeping noise is.

The suite was large and comfortable, but clearly hadn't been used for sleeping. There were stacks of paper everywhere. The room had floor to ceiling windows that were thrown open revealing spectacular views of the Mediterranean. There were three men waiting on us. Two got up to welcome me, and the third remained seated. He looked gruff. He never looked up; he just barked, 'Seat... sit.'

They spoke French with a smattering of English. 'Sit ... come ... pace'. I spoke German, but don't know a word of French beyond the expected salutations. I didn't know what to say so I muttered, '*Bonjour.*' That went over like a lead balloon.

There was a faint smell of tobacco in the room, which probably accounted for the windows being wide open or perhaps it was a lack of air conditioning. Either way, the air was simmering with tension. The scene would have been complete had one of the three actually pulled out a cigarette.

It was probably just as well that they didn't speak much English because judging from their faces they were in no humour for indolence. One of them asked, 'What's the problem, O'Mara?'

I blurted, 'Look, I don't mean to be difficult, but I really have no interest in this pacing job.'

One of the other two promptly interjected with something along the lines of, 'Saïd wants you. He says you do a good job.'

'That's nice, but I really would prefer not to.'

The director muttered something in French and motioned his hands impatiently. The English speaker interpreted for me. 'We will pay $6,000 plus a bonus.'

I just shook my head, declining with a simple, 'No.'

The French spoke among themselves while I shifted in my seat nervously.

I felt more resolution than my solitary presence suggested. I attempted to explain that I had run 3:52 and was aiming for a national record. Clearly no one cared beyond the fact that it suggested that I had the wheels to run fast for three laps. They continued nattering as if I wasn't even there.

The chatter stopped, and the English speaker said, 'We are going to offer you $8,000.'

'I am really sorry. I just have no interest in pacing,' I retorted.

Another conclave was held, a little more heated this time, more volume, more animation. Suddenly the director turns to me and holds up ten fingers. Had I just been offered $10,000 to pace a mile? Yes, I had and judging by the contented look on his face, he was certain he had hit the sweet spot. Shockingly for him, my position didn't change. I held fast to my principles. I trained all year to pursue my goals, not someone else's.

Eventually, I was offered $12,000. Before I could refuse once again, the director grabbed a wad of $100 bills from his briefcase which was sitting slightly open on the floor alongside him. He laid out twelve stacks of ten-dollar bills in a fan shape before me, robotically counting each hundred of every thousand and every thousand. One hundred, two hundred, three hundred … one thousand, all the way to twelve thousand. Then he stood up to amplify the moment.

He read my eyes and instantly surmised that I was going to reject this offer too. I wasn't immune to the temptation. It was a whole lot of money, still is, but my decision was firm. His frustration turned to anger. They were done negotiating with themselves.

I can't remember the words he employed because it was in very broken English. Either I took the $12,000 and set the pace, or I would be sent home without having set foot on the track. The math had changed. It was no longer $12,000 versus $3,000. Now it was twelve versus zero.

I didn't flinch. If I succumbed to the pressure, I would never shake off the pacemaker tag, forever labelled as inauthentic, a second-class athlete. I knew the answer intuitively and said, 'I am so sorry. I've been telling you the whole time that I am simply not interested.'

All eyes were glaring at me and a couple right through me. Then he simply dismissed me with a curt, 'Leave!'

I looked back over my shoulder as I left the room to see the director hurriedly gathering up what could have been mine.

A little while later the phone in my room rang, and it was the junior director. Apparently, when Saïd was told about my refusal, he instructed the meeting director to reinstate me. He never wanted me to be bullied into submission. The Irish record was still a go that night.

The irony is my good friend, Ray Flynn, was engaged to make the pace. This could have meant that he paced a fellow country man to break his

Irish record. Ray gambled well. I had a good run, but it wasn't a special night. I was third in 3:53.60. Unfortunately for Ray and Saïd, they missed the world record. I never asked Ray how much he was paid for his effort, but I know he got the last laugh that weekend.

I was hounded for the remainder of the year with pace-making requests and capitulated to Enrico's persistence at season's end. Saïd planned a world record attempt in the 2,000m at the Van Damme meeting in Brussels. Saïd had been a good ally and wielded a lot of influence. Plus, I kind of owed him one. I pulled him through a mile in 3:54. Saïd ran 4:51.98 and barely missed the world record 4:51.35. I hit my marks, and the universe was back in equilibrium. I was excused from further pace-making duties.

I have always lived by the imprimatur, if you stand for nothing you will fall for anything. Well, I stood up for myself in the face of temptation. I showed resolve when I rejected the biggest sum of money I had ever seen. Of course, I failed to break our national record, but I still think I made the right decision for the right reasons. I had clear and tangible reasons to believe I could run under 3:50. I had just completed three times 800m in 1:50, 1:50 and 1:51 in training, ample evidence that I was very fit.

It was the absence of evidence that caused me to re-evaluate my commitment to the pulsing protocol. Without a doubt, there were elements of legitimacy at the beginning. After all, people are regularly cured of Lyme disease. It is the chronic version that requires a leap of faith.

It took two years total for me to wise up and connect the dots. The disciplined approach I had relied on so extensively had vanished, overwhelmed by an ability to persevere, driven by a burning desire to shake off Parkinson's. When I finally opened my eyes and catalogued the evidence to support this treatment, there wasn't much to see. There simply wasn't a

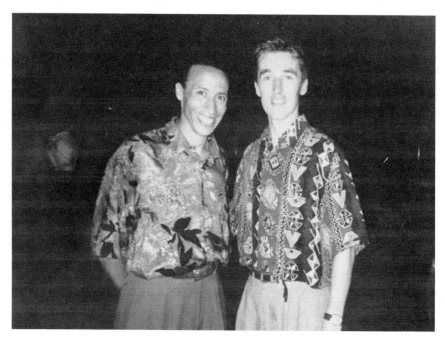

August 1987. Matching shirts with Saïd Aouita.

single data point propping up a continuance.

Initially, I felt an overwhelming sense of foolishness. I always prided myself on pragmatism and have always had a reasonable nonsense detector, but each failed me miserably. Then there was the element of shame. I had clearly embarrassed myself with the whole affair, but I especially felt for Patty. She supported my decision to stay the course when I know many of her friends appealed to her to intercede. Finally, I was sad. Sad because I couldn't undo the misjudgement. It's not the same as taking a wrong turn while using GPS. There is no 'recalibrating' an alternate route; you have permanently veered off course and you are headed toward a whole new set of issues. I had to accept the finality of the mistake to move on. The blame was mine alone.

In the end, I was too distracted with coping on an hourly basis to wallow in shame. I vowed to learn from this mishap just as I had from a slew of athletic disappointments. It was high time to acknowledge that I should never have left the care of Dr Archer and UAMS. Apologies were in order.

## CHAPTER 10

# DON'T LOOK BEYOND YOUR HEADLIGHTS

I had not seen Dr Archer in over two years. I was compunctious about the absence and couldn't blame him if he declined to renew our doctor-patient relationship. It's not easy making amends, especially to an expert who happened to have been correct all along. I wrote him a heartfelt email of apology.

He was more than pleased to see me. He understood why I had pursued the Lyme treatment and he remarked, 'I couldn't offer you as much hope. However slim the odds were, I don't blame you for pursuing it.'

I told him about the saga and described how worn out I was from all the antibiotics. He listened intently and asked, 'How many Sinemet are you currently taking?'

Sinemet is not a panacea for Parkinson's. It doesn't cure, not even temporarily, it just makes coping more manageable. I had called Dr Archer's office during the height of the antibiotic onslaught asking for the flexibility to take extra should my condition warrant it. He gladly obliged and I had *carte blanche* over daily consumption.

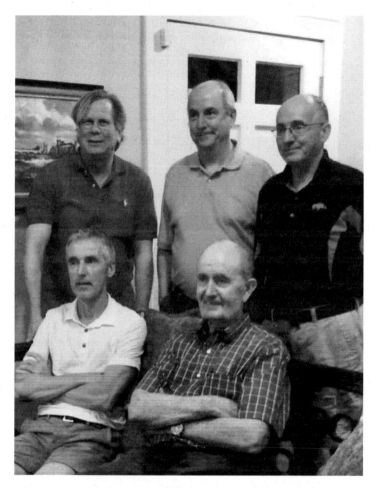

Standing (L-R) Dr Mark Andersen (who was on that run where I experienced my first symptom), Dr Archer, Niall O'Shaughnessy. Seated: Me and my coach, John McDonnell.

I answered, 'Ten, and closer to twelve.' Determined to be completely honest, I admitted, 'Actually, it's twelve on a good day.'

To me, the increase in Sinemet is an indication of how much I had retreated in the battle with Parkinson's. During my hiatus from neurological care, a long two years, I had doubled my intake. Unfortunately, there are side effects to too much Sinemet: dyskinesia and jerkiness. I was now in the danger zone and was experiencing more than my fair share of unwanted movements. In the lost two years, I missed the innovative use of agonists, which would have enabled a lower dosage of Sinemet. Agonists stimulate the dopamine receptors in the brain and mimic the effects of dopamine allowing lower dosages of the primary drug. Delayed release versions of agonists have been particularly helpful and ultimately would have a major impact on my wellbeing.

I was entirely dependent by now, and I sometimes wondered how badly I would feel if I was ever deprived of Sinemet. Sure, I had missed a dose by a couple of hours, but what about an extended period?

I unwittingly discovered how dependent I was on Sinemet on a return trip from New York City. It was a baking hot afternoon, and we were over-dressed and sweaty by the time the taxi dropped us at the terminal. We only had carry-on baggage and made it through the TSA line just in time to board our plane to Atlanta.

We were no sooner on board than the captain notified us of bad weather in the Carolinas, but he was hopeful that the weather pattern would have moved through by the time we arrived. His hopefulness was misplaced. After we pushed back from the gate with the help of a tug and before the captain could even start the engines, he informed us that we had to be towed back to the terminal. Traffic Control advised that the weather in Atlanta was deteriorating and would be too unstable when we were expected to land. We were in a holding pattern.

Then the captain announced, 'There are no gates available so we will remain parked for the moment.' Well, it was much more than a moment.

We remained parked on the apron. Critically, there was no air conditioning since the engines were not running. We sat in the torrid sun as the temperature began rising inside the metal fuselage. The captain urged us to lower all window shades in a futile attempt to fight the increasing heat. Flight attendants frantically handed out ice water. The heat kept building as passengers began removing shoes and socks, shirts were unbuttoned, men stripped down to undershirts. Women didn't have that luxury, mind you some must have been tempted.

Then it dawned on me. Did I bring extra medication? I quickly pulled my mini ziplock baggie from my jacket pocket and began counting. Then I re-counted. If I managed to get home tonight, I had one more dose than needed. However, the trauma of sitting in this motorised tin can could make me symptomatic, and I could easily consume the extra dose just to survive. And what if we missed our connection in Atlanta? The heat kept rising like a pork shoulder on a smoker, slowly but surely.

I turned to Patty and asked, 'What are the chances that you brought back-up medicine in your purse?'

I already knew the reply. 'Only headache pills. What do you need?'

I explained my dilemma and she advised, 'You can't be sure we won't make the connection, and you're suffering now. I'd take the extra if you need it.'

Not long after, I began to shake and became extremely restless. The escalating heat and the close confines of the cabin drove me to consume my meagre insurance policy. Ultimately, we sat on the runway for over an hour. Tempers were frayed, nerves were frazzled, but finally we were towed back to an open gate where we were connected to power and the miracle of air conditioning was rediscovered.

After a further two hours waiting for the weather to clear, we were on our way. Our arrival time was anticipated to be well past midnight, long after our last connection to Little Rock. With the day now extended past 1:00am, I was forced to take my last dose. I was miserable when we got to Atlanta at 12:35am, having exhausted my supply of Sinemet. It was clear that I was going to have a rough time sleeping so best to catch the early flight in the morning and limit the misery. We had to queue at customer service to make alternate flight arrangements and again to wait for transfer to a nearby hotel. It was 2:00am by the time our heads hit the pillow. I was shaky, but managed to survive. Tomorrow would be a different challenge.

A paltry few hours later, the alarm rattled us from sleep. Without my morning allocation of Sinemet, I immediately felt the Parkinson's symptoms overwhelm me. It was going to be an arduous morning, and I steeled myself for the check-in line, the TSA line, the line to board. There would be nowhere to hide. I waited for the shuttle bus in the lobby, and I was glad to see we were the only passengers in the van. I was visibly shaking and uncoordinated as I flopped into the front row. My walking was ungainly at best. Patty had downloaded the boarding passes, and we slowly headed for the TSA line. To our surprise, at 6:00am, the TSA was awash with other travellers. Some were business travellers, some were vacationers, some dressed well, some dressed like they were about to spend the night on a friend's sofa. I was intimidated by the throngs. The line inched forward as I barely clung to my task.

Patty persuaded me that I could cope. 'Nobody here knows you, who cares how you look?' she said.

'But they are all staring at me. I can tell.'

I was the morning entertainment, and I could tell that people were wondering, *What's up with your man?*

It must have taken thirty minutes as we wound our way through the labyrinth and that was in the pre-check lane. We managed somehow and made our way to the train to take us to Terminal B. The train was standing room only with the exception of a couple of disabled seats at the ends of the carriage. My legs were unstable and tired, and I was looking forward to sitting in one of those seats. To my dismay, the seats were occupied by a couple of young girls. I hate playing the crippled card, so I gripped tightly to the bar. The swaying of the carriage disguised much of the shaking. The train and I appeared to move in concert.

We ploughed on and eventually made it to the gate. Patty plonked me in the disabled seating. I recognised some faces of others heading to Little Rock, but nobody in my circle of acquaintances. I sat, not very still mind you, and waited impatiently to board. I closed my eyes and began a deep breathing routine. There was no dozing off, however. My body was out of control. I was gyrating in the chair. Boarding brought no great comfort. I was boxed in on a commuter jet, no leg room and no arm room and no head room. Fortunately, Patty is not a large person, and her reassuring words helped me find an internal peace.

'We are almost there now. The worst is behind us,' she said.

The worst was well behind us, and we made it home safely, but not unblemished. It was a frightening experience. I was exhausted from all the stress and body motion. We made a pact never to repeat the experience. I now bring double the required medicine for every trip even if that requires a vacation override from my health insurance provider, and Patty always has an emergency stash in her purse.

I had become so dependent that missing one dose had turned my world upside down. I wondered what would happen if my body ever became immune to the liberating effect of the drug. Could the ever-increasing dosage harm the effectiveness? Should I fight the urge to increase the amount?

It seems simple enough. You are fighting against a regressive disease, so it stands to reason that as time progresses your brain produces ever decreasing levels of dopamine. But the side effect to excessive amounts of Sinemet was equally disturbing – the nuisance known as dyskinesia. It could be head nodding, it could be torso swaying, it could be twitchy legs. For me, it was all of the above.

Dyskinesia renders you incapable of doing simple tasks. I remember on many occasions sitting in front of the computer to answer emails. The keyboard was at the optimal height, and the seat correctly positioned. I was ergonomically primed. Confronting the keyboard, I deployed a manoeuvre that involved my torso snapping from right to left and at the correct moment my right arm would dart south, and my index finger would tap a key. Then on the return trip, the left arm would perform a similar move. Needless to say, my email responses were extremely succinct and often riddled with misspellings.

Dealing with balance issues can be a harrowing experience too. Simple tasks like balancing on one leg while you lift the other to dress yourself became impossible. I learned to manage by leaning against a wall to provide a backstop, which doesn't work on a wooden floor if you are in socks. Of course, there is always the option to sit, but I had trouble keeping my balance while seated. Somehow, I ended up on my side in the crunch position. Worse yet, if I chose a seat without sides, like an ottoman or a bench, I could find myself lying on the ground.

Parkinson's is a movement disorder, so it is no wonder that walking issues became a major problem. Given that my first symptom was ambulation, severe gait issues were even more predictable for me. My walking was dreadful. It was unpleasant to both watch and endure. I could get from A to B, but I frequently took a more scenic route.

There appeared to be four different varieties based on time of day and Sinemet levels. The first I labelled 'High Step.' This style was characterised by needless vertical motion with little horizontal progress; high knees and heavy stomping were its main features.

The second category I called 'Lurch'. The star of this show was the upper body, which seemed in a hurry to get somewhere while my legs showed no

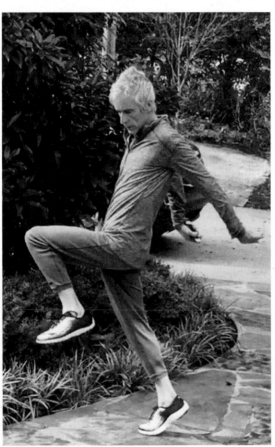

The 'high step' walk.

interest in following, leaving me leaning forward, chest almost parallel to the ground. This was dangerous because of the high risk of falling.

The next was 'Pinball', distinctive for its total lack of control. I barrelled down hallways ricocheting off walls, slamming into doors or walls to stop or clinging onto door jambs to redirect. Twice I have indented the sheetrock in our home by crashing into walls. I marvel at how strong my fingers are from gripping a 1cm lip on a countertop or door moulding. Everyone who spends time in our house knows that the first five centimetres of every flat surface has to be kept clear so that I can use it for guidance or stability. With this method there is also a high risk of falls or of knocking things over.

The fourth variety is 'Penguin'. It's not pretty, but it's the best available to me. Like a penguin, I don't swing my arms, they lie dormant by my side. My back is stiff, and I wobble from side to side. It also features a knee that rolls in and hyper extends, but I can make progress.

It's a strange feeling when you consider walking an achievement. Even more strange when you catch yourself showing off your clumsy ability. I once prided myself on the speed of my running. Now I am like a parent thrilled over a child's first steps.

If I could predict when the Penguin was due to appear, I could commit to attending events and simply getting out of the house.

I knew there were periods of most days when I felt relatively normal. Although those windows were constantly shrinking, if I could just identify when they would be most likely to occur, I could plan. I needed to account for every hour of every day to identify any trend or aggregation of good periods. I created an Excel sheet to track medications and how I felt every hour throughout the day. Each hour was labelled either Green (Okay),

Orange (Poor) or Red (Awful). I tracked every waking hour and noted the quality of the previous night's sleep. When I didn't feel well enough to enter the data, I wrote on the closest piece of paper and uploaded it later. I still find random pieces of paper laying around the house with notations like '3-4 orange' or '4-5 green'.

The monthly data allowed me to identify segments of time when I was most likely to feel good and most importantly make social commitments. It was a chore and required a certain degree of obsession, but I kept these hour-by-hour records for the next four years. I produced graphs that illustrated trends and provided my doctors with meaningful feedback.

In my case, there was a considerable increase of Sinemet in the background and ever-growing propagation of red on the chart. It was a sad barometer of my decline since the last time I had been in Dr Archer's offices.

He had read my email and knew I had been chastened and even a little humbled. He had been copied by the Lyme doctor on all appointment recaps and knew I had been through the wars. We discussed next steps, and then Dr Archer revealed that he had hired a Movement Disorder Specialist and would like him to take over my care.

That was fantastic news. I had read about these specialists and had considered asking for a referral.

'Tell me more about him,' I eagerly inquired.

He proceeded to lay out Dr Dhall's experience. It was impressive. Among his previous roles was the directorship of the Parkinson's Foundation Center of Excellence at the Muhammad Ali Medical Center in Arizona. He had authored numerous articles on Parkinson's and led multiple research efforts.

Dr Archer next reminded me of advice he had previously given me that I should consider deep brain stimulation (DBS). 'I've told Dr Dhall that you're an excellent candidate for implants, but I want him to exhaust everything in his arsenal before we go to that extreme.'

I was curious what techniques might obviate the need for brain surgery, which I was in no hurry to consider. Trying not to highlight the fact that I'd taken a two-year hiatus from treatment, I responded, 'What techniques have we not tried?'

'There are agonists we haven't tried and various experimental trials you can be a part of. Don't worry, deep brain stimulation will be a last resort,' Dr Archer informed me.

The reality that I was a candidate for deep brain stimulation alarmed me, but I would need to be really desperate to submit to that ordeal. I had learned from previous experiences – all of my journeys through boarding school, running, moving abroad – that when faced with a daunting task, you need to understand your options completely. Fully explore each before you allow someone to hook you up to the power grid. I had to inventory available options.

When you are fighting an insidious disease like Parkinson's you must adopt a day-to-day approach. Incrementalise to the smallest degree, day by day if possible, or even hour by hour.

You cannot look beyond your headlights. Get up, put on your armour and engage in combat. Whatever the disease throws at you, on any particular day, you need to be prepared. Whether it is freezing, gait issues, a fall, speech problems, all you can give is your best.

If I dwelled on future battles, on next year's disease presentation, I would be crippled with fear.

So, I ameliorate the dread by giving each day my best effort. When I close my eyes at night, I know I gave Parkinson's a run for its money that day. I focus on the now to the exclusion of yesterday and especially tomorrow.

If the plan is to ignore past and future, then you need an accurate assessment of the present. The colour-coded sheets told the true story. I discovered that I hadn't been honest with myself or indeed with others, including my medical team. I made sure I only spent time outside the house when I had the maximum likelihood of feeling okay. If my condition was less than it ought to be at the anointed hour, I invariably cancelled. It's strange how determined I was to only appear when I was in optimum shape. Even on visits with my neurologist, the one person I surely couldn't fool, I put my best foot forward.

Dr Dhall loved the reams of legal-sized papers adorned with coloured cells. The data provided a rapid and reliable feedback loop on the different drug protocols we tried. He was particularly careful not to contaminate the results. He was more deliberate than circumspect. He made one change at a time, so it was imperative that we had the fastest, most accurate feedback possible. Dr Dhall was trying to determine if there was a cocktail of medicine that might obviate the necessity of surgery.

Since Sinemet is the primary workhorse, all other drugs must work in symphony with it. The only question was would an agonist, such as Amantadine, improve Sinemet's efficacy. The primary agonist that Dr Dhall wished to experiment with was a drug called Rytary. He had seen tremendous success with numerous other patients and hoped for a similar response from me. Unfortunately, my reaction was entirely different. A quick perusal of the colour-coded chart told its own tale, way too much red. We abandoned that change promptly.

Parkinson's consumed me. I thought about it all day. Although it was sometimes quiet, it regularly erupted. It was my constant companion. My every conversation somehow managed to include the dastardly topic. I was in a constant struggle, and I had little else to talk about.

I always felt I had a little storyteller in me – most Irish people do – but now I had so little material to work with. I had allowed my interests to dwindle and my friends to decline through lack of energy and poor health. I knew that I must fight lethargy and stay engaged.

## CHAPTER 11

# TAKE RESPONSIBILITY

Parkinson's is an odious foe. Just when you feel you have learned to cope with a particular line of attack, it assaults another crucial function. I had begun to experience swallowing challenges and had a few mild scares digesting food. Of course, there was an accompanying annoyance ... drooling. The subtle kind that you hardly notice until your shirt collar is a pool of dampness. Even more troublesome then either of these, my speech was now barely audible or understandable.

On a visit to Dr Dhall, he said, 'Your speech has become very hypophonic.'

'I haven't heard that term before. To me, my voice feels breathy.'

Parkinson's can affect the vocal cords and leave insufficient breath to speak. When you speak, air moves from your lungs over your vocal cords which vibrate and produce speech. In Parkinson's patients, the muscle of the cord becomes thinner and less taut, causing them to lose shape and no longer close properly. This creates a gap which allows air to escape, and softness or hoarseness can result.

I had noticed that, try as I might, one breath delivered fewer words. I felt I was gulping for air midway through a sentence. Additionally, I noticed that whatever breath I did take was really shallow. A breath seemed to stay in the airways, almost in the throat. I described the sensation to Dr Dhall.

He listened and remarked, 'We have excellent speech therapists at UAMS, and I believe they can help you with volume.'

Therapy consisted of what amounted to be shouting exercises. When I practised at home our dog scurried from the room each time. I mentioned this to the therapist, she measured my volume on a sound metre, and what seemed to be shouting to me barely registered as noise. So, we also worked on breathing and lung depletion.

I had an appointment with a specialist about vocal-cord augmentation. She described three procedures that increased in complexity as benefit duration climbed. She suggested that we begin with the temporary version, and let the results determine the next steps.

The doctor administered shots of silicon directly into the vocal cords. This plumped up the cords and enabled them to retain breath and push out the words with greater volume.

'How long will the benefit last?' I asked.

'It should last two to three months.' She carried on, 'If that works, we'll schedule you for a more permanent procedure.'

I was encouraged by my response to the shots. The volume of my voice improved, but the improvement lasted little more than the expected couple of months. I immediately contacted the doctor to schedule the semi-permanent procedure. I was keen to address the problem promptly as the last few weeks of near-adequate conversation had felt like a luxury. I had to wait a month to get a surgery date, and in the meantime, my voice therapist made an interesting suggestion that might eliminate the need for surgery.

The device was called SpeechVive, and it was designed to fake the user into speaking louder. The concept was simple but clever and was inspired by a natural human response to talking in a crowded room. The noisier the room becomes, the louder you are forced to speak. If the ambient noise levels increase, your voice automatically adjusts. The creators developed an earbud that plays a compilation of simultaneous conversations to simulate a crowded room. The conversations are indeterminable and serve only as a volume hurdle that you have to overcome to be heard. The clever bit is the background noise ceases once you begin speaking and reinitiates once you stop. It definitely gives you the sensation of shouting.

I tried the device on multiple occasions. It did have its merits, but it wasn't for me. Listening to that racket all day would have driven me insane. Plus, it was twenty times more expensive than my Apple earbuds and would likely become the costliest thing I'd ever mislay or accidentally run through the washing machine.

About six weeks later I had vocal-cord augmentation surgery in Little Rock. My doctor placed implants in my larynges. The procedure lasted little under an hour and the substance she implanted was dissolvable and eventually would break down. I saw a marked improvement in my volume for a time, but as predicted the benefit didn't last.

There is a permanent solution that I haven't availed myself of yet. Based on the positive outcome of the temporary solutions, it would likely help. The question is would it help during an Off Period when I am entombed in fatigue and indifference and cannot muster the energy to be heard?

More concerning, I have developed a cognitive speech issue. When a topic is simple or a conversation one-dimensional, my voice is fine. For example, a response to an enquiry about how you are doing doesn't take much processing power. It could be as simple as, 'Great, thanks.' The answer does not require much effort to formulate.

Conversely, if asked to describe the merits of indexed mutual funds, I'd have to devote more effort to explain. There are multiple parts that must be assembled in the background, in the correct sequence for your reply to make sense. A normally functioning brain processes the answer in a micro-second and continues to formulate as you respond. My brain just displays a twirling hourglass. I may begin adequately, but by the time 'dollar cost averaging' gets a mention, my response very quickly turns to garbage.

Sometimes, when I feel I might give in, and can't muster the energy to take part in life, I think of people who have inspired me in various ways. I had a very good friend from secondary school who turned into quite a role model. He was perhaps the most sensible man I have ever met. His name was Niall O'Shaughnessy. He was a boarder and was four years ahead of me at St Munchin's. He held all our school's middle-distance records.

Three years before Niall, another St Munchin's pupil, Neil Cusack, left his mark on the intercollegiate track circuit. Neil became the first Irishman to win the NCAA Cross Country Championships in 1973 and won the Boston Marathon in 1974. I admired Neil and was overawed when he acknowledged me at practice in the LPYMA grounds, a grass track we trained on in Limerick. There was a massive roller with a harness attached so a horse could pull it around the track to smooth the surface. We didn't have a horse, so the bigger lads would reluctantly drag the roller around.

One evening as the seniors were attempting to get momentum going on the roller, Neil spotted me and said, 'Hey you, O'Mara! Get over here with some of your pals and help us pull this damn thing.' He acknowledged me, so that was a plus!

Niall and Neil both made the Irish Olympic team in 1976 in Montreal.

They set a very high bar for those of us who follow in their footsteps. I overlapped at St Munchin's with Niall by a year, and I was especially fond of him. A few years later, Father MacNamee, the school president, invited me to the staff quarters one evening to watch Niall race in the Wanamaker Mile at the Madison Square Gardens, where he took on Dick Buerkle. The previous weekend in Missouri, Niall had run the second fastest indoor mile ever. We were all exceptionally proud to watch a schoolmate excel in the crucible of modern professional sport, the Madison Square Gardens.

Niall has always been a talisman for me, and I mimicked his every move. When I saw him in red suede Puma racing shoes, I had to have a pair. I followed him to the University of Arkansas. I studied civil engineering just like he did, and I lived in the same dormitory. During my freshman year he showed me, in his quiet way, how to apply myself, how to cope with being so far from home and how to juggle school and athletics. I ignored his advice to pursue, as he had, a master's in civil engineering, and instead chose the less arduous master's in business administration.

He was principled, almost to a fault. He withdrew from consideration for the Irish Olympic team for the 1980 games in Moscow. The USA had boycotted the Russian Olympics because of their invasion of Afghanistan and Niall, who had just received his master's in engineering with the full intention of working in the United States and becoming a citizen, elected not to compete in solidarity.

We kept in touch over the years. He called after he heard I had Parkinson's, and I could feel the wisdom in his advice as he once again counselled me on how to cope when you are in over your head. A few years later, while suffering through largely difficult days, I received a call from our old coach.

Niall had been diagnosed with a brain tumour. I dropped the phone in disbelief! How could a bloke, who had never done anyone a bad turn, be so afflicted? Not that bad happens exclusively to bad people, but Niall was one of the truly good guys.

Once I had picked myself up off the floor, I dialled Niall's number, and he picked up. I led with, 'Niall, I am so sorry to hear the news.'

The reply was the usual positive Niall. 'It will be alright, I'm in good hands at the hospital.'

'Have you figured out your care plan?' I asked.

'My brother, David, is trying to get me into a hospital that specialises in my kind of situation,' he went on, before he described the general plan of attack.

Then he enquired about my health. 'How have you been doing?'

'You know how it is, Niall. Some days are bad, and some are not so bad.' After some more banter, namely about the medical profession and how invaluable they had become in both our lives, he said, 'I'll tell you something, Frank. I'd much rather be me than you. Either I get better, or I don't. You're never going to get better.'

'But I get to live.'

'And deteriorate every year.'

'I'm not so sure, Niall.'

It was an extraordinarily candid interaction and one that illustrates his pragmatic side.

Coincidentally, a little while later we were at dinner in Fayetteville, and Patty was sitting beside Niall. Late in the evening, Niall leaned into Patty and whispered, 'Take care of Frank; he is worse off than me.' He was entirely selfless. And Patty assured me that she answered, 'I will.'

Niall died a little more than a year later. John McDonnell and I flew to Atlanta to say goodbye around three weeks before he passed away. We also presented him with a medal inducting him into the Southwest Conference Sports Hall of Fame for his remarkable college athletics career.

I remember Niall often in my daily struggles and hope I am living with some level of the dignity that he would display if he was in my shoes. I have my cross to bear, but I am in the land of the living. The courage and selflessness he exhibited are my guiding light.

* * *

Nighttime can be scary for many afflicted with Parkinson's. On this account, I have a pretty clean record, specifically, when it comes to staying in bed for the duration of the night. However, getting into bed and calming my body down so that I could sleep was like folding a fitted sheet, close to impossible.

First, getting on the bed was enormously difficult. I approached it like I was about to mount a horse. One hand ready to peel back the covers and the other to use as leverage as I swung my legs onto the bed and hoped that I landed in a comfortable position. This move requires multiple commands. One to each arm and one queued up for my legs. The required coordination confused my brain and impounded my body. The mind said 'go' but couldn't complete the transmission. Invariably I ended up frozen in place as I confronted the obstacle, my hour-clock spinning wildly at the impasse. A gentle nudge from Patty was needed to break the sequence. We came up with a workaround. Patty would take my hand and lead me around the bedroom like a horse being led around the parade ring before a race. This manoeuvre essentially reset my brain, however temporarily.

'Clear your mind now,' she would advise, to which I would mutter affirmatively. The routine was to suddenly peel off and immediately leap onto the bed.

'Come on now, first time,' she encouraged. 'You can do it!'

I suddenly peeled off, and with a total lack of grace managed to get on the bed. The art was not in the execution of the move itself but in the final placement. Once on the bed I was done. Whatever position I ended up with had better be satisfactory.

She always asked, 'Are you good like that?'

Invariably I wasn't ideally positioned for sleep. In truth no position was ideal because of my inability to relax. I also lacked the capacity to self-adjust. To provide some assurance that a particular position was acceptable, I practised sleeping positions during the day. These simulations were essential at bedtime to help soothe my doubts. It was a mind game that I have a losing record in. Many nights it took multiple attempts.

Those times when I couldn't manage, I simply started over.

'Patty, help!'

'You need to start over?'

Back to the parade ring again, hoping for a more accurate landing. Eventually, I would get satisfactorily situated and allow deep breathing to finally take control. Amazingly, one full breath makes a dent, and three consecutive breaths quell the incessant shaking. If I can get five full breaths, consecutive without disturbance, I am asleep.

For me, a freezing episode always seems to involve multiple tasks at once. A classic example is brushing my teeth. Leaning over the sink, one hand moving the toothbrush, the other hand on the tap requires three commands, turn the tap, lean, brush. I often stand over the sink for an eternity, motionless, trying to let go of the tap or turn off the electric toothbrush that has been twirling away and often splashing toothpaste on the mirror like a NutriBullet. The more I try to complete the task, the more stubborn the resistance becomes.

Lately, I have devised a technique to combat freezing. It's a little counterintuitive. It involves introducing a new and unassociated action to break the cycle. If instead of attempting to turn off the brush, I decided to drop it in the sink, and that same instant dropped it, then the handbrake would be released. Similarly, with getting into bed at night, if I decided to squat down rather than the intended spring forward, I would be freed of incapacity. The decision and action must be simultaneous. There can be no deliberation. I have a series of tricks that I alternate. Parkinson's is a wily foe and figures out your charade. Then I move on to the next option. I rotate through my options regularly and I practise these schemes when I am well, so they are natural when deployed.

Once settled, I am shocked at how I manage to sleep relatively well given my proclivity to shake when woken. With Parkinson's, it is very troublesome to make subconscious adjustments in position. I wake with some frequency to adjust, and I rely on the miracle of deep breathing to get through those adventures too.

I haven't always been that fortunate. I have been a bad sleeper as far back as I can remember. My mother told stories of my father taking me to my bedroom to put me to sleep. The house completely silent in case the toddler was distracted. She would hear the bedroom door creak open and try to decipher if she heard adult or kid footsteps creeping back toward the living room. Invariably, it was the short shuffling of a child. I would peep round the door. My father was asleep.

In boarding school, I was a dormitory prefect. Each of the dormitories had an oversized cubicle in which the prefect slept. The prefect was expected to maintain control, especially after lights out, watch out for illness and basically monitor the younger pupils. I was assigned to the first-year dormitory. Maintaining discipline wasn't a challenge; the problem was loneliness. You were separated from your friends and family and living with a bunch of eleven-year-olds.

I don't know what came first, the loneliness or the sleeplessness. I do know that I would lie in bed for hours. Frequently, I got up and roamed the corridors, dark as winter in the polar regions. On occasion, I would step into the phone kiosk and pick up the handset, wait for the dial tone and quietly dial my home number. My intention – my wish – was that my parents would come to get me, save me from the place.

I never completed a call. It was often well after midnight, and I didn't want to alarm my parents. That struggle went on for the entire year that I was imbedded with the eleven-year-olds and left an indelible mark on me. I wish I had known then that I could combat problems using breathing techniques, but perhaps I wouldn't have agreed to the cost of that lesson, having learned it courtesy of Parkinson's.

Although I was at times unhappy, St Munchin's was by and large a positive experience. At the very least it was a highly formative one. Separated from my family, I became independent, and I developed good communications skills. At my core, I tend toward introversion, like my mother, but I also share some of my father's jocosity. I've always had that dichotomy of extroversion versus introversion and was often accused of being moody in school. I imagine the battle between these inclinations is responsible for my on-off relationship with boarding school. It certainly explains the moodiness.

There is no denying we had some funny and very memorable experiences in boarding school. One of those events is well worth describing.

Adherence to protocol and schedule were crucial elements of maintaining discipline and the morning rituals were particularly rigorous. The first bell rang rudely at 6:10am signalling that you had twenty minutes to be dressed and downstairs in your assigned seat in the chapel for mass. This bell was routinely ignored, except for the diligent few who practised good dental hygiene. The second bell was ten minutes later and this one was generally complied with. You had just about enough time to take care of the basics and make it to church on time, but there was no room for a hiccup. There was a further bell which garnered impressive support, and this one allowed a mere five minutes.

One of our friends was the dormitory prefect for the fourth years and one day complained about what a slothful group his charges were. No matter how hard he tried to rouse them in the morning they slept until the third bell. Then it was a mad charge to get dressed and sprint through the corridors to church. Don't bother with the teeth. We channelled our inner Shackleton and decided a lesson in discipline was appropriate.

The plan was simple but would require careful execution. If these dilletantes got up at the five-minute bell and couldn't find their trousers, wouldn't that be hilarious? The panic they would feel at the prospect of being late for mass was worth any repercussion. The key is we'd have to get every pair, otherwise we would just cause an inconvenience. It would take effort and time to search for other trousers beyond the one recently discarded and lying in immediate view on the back of the chair. Thankfully, there were very few options, one tiny closet and an equally unimpressive space for a bag under the bed and of course in plain view draped over a skinny metal chair with wood veneer finish.

Alarm clocks were verboten, so the six of us involved in this escapade took turns staying awake. We took thirty-minute shifts before handing the post off to the next person. At two in the morning, the last watch woke the others, and we hastily reviewed the plan. We had divided the dormitory into areas of equal size, each person responsible for removing any trousers found in the cubicle. Expediency was paramount and there was to be no searching beyond the three likely spots. After separating the trousers from its owner, you would carry your ever-growing bundle from cubicle to cubicle. When it became too cumbersome, we left the pile on the floor to be gathered later.

Our hearts pounded as we opened the large wooden door which we knew would creak. We opened it slowly which only served to elongate the sound and created a slow-motion version of eeeeeeeeekkkkkk. We froze mid-action and held our breath, convinced we'd woken the entire building. All we heard was the gentle breathing of fifty or so boys. We had dispensed with slippers in favour of socks, and we crept gently by each cubicle to our designated area. As I slinked past one cubicle, the occupant partially rose up and stared at me. It startled me, but we had anticipated this scenario. I simply put my index finger to my lips and whispered, 'It's alright. Go back to sleep.' Oddly, he complied.

Once we were in position, we silently pillaged every trouser we could find. We moved our piles along as we progressed and ended up with a mound by the door. We were in pure stealth mode, like ninjas. None of the sleeping souls woke, but we still had to open the door one more time and keep it ajar until the pile had been relocated into the corridor. From there the plan was to stash the pile in the last cubicle in the nuns' bathroom. We laboured mightily to transport our swag down a flight of stairs to the sisters' wing. The procurement and logistics exercise over, we returned to our beds to wait for the ructions that were certain to erupt.

We were up at the first bell, anxious to see how our prank would be viewed. We tried our best to seem uninterested as we passed the dormitory on our way to the chapel. There appeared to be no movement; they were, as anticipated, waiting for the five-minute bell. In church, there was a designated section for each school year; as we slid into our area, we noticed that there wasn't a single individual in the entire fourth year area. Stragglers rolled in, but there wasn't a fourth year among them. Suddenly, the gravity of what we had done became apparent. The sacristy door opened, and the priest walked to the altar flanked by two altar boys. When he turned to face the school, he immediately noticed a large empty section of the church.

There were six missing rows. He came down from the altar and stood on the parquet floor of the sanctuary and asked if anyone knew how an entire class could be missing. Nobody knew anything except the six of us, and we weren't speaking anytime soon.

He removed his vestments to reveal his black suit and dog collar. There is something intimidating about that look. He handed the vestments to an altar boy and stormed off. To his dismay, he didn't find a problem with the alarm or a bunch of oversleeping kids. Instead, he found kids wandering around in their underwear or pyjamas totally unsure what they ought to do next. A massive search of the dormitory was apparently carried out which revealed nothing. The remainder of the school body waited anxiously in the chapel. Everyone speculated on what had just happened and who may be responsible. Talking was not allowed in church, so there was a lot of whispering and muttering. Suddenly, the rear doors flung open, and the dean was back from the scene of the crime. He demanded to know who the culprits were. If they didn't confess, the entire student body would suffer the consequences.

Before he could describe what assortment of punishment he had in mind, one of the nuns appeared and summoned the dean. A large stash of male clothing had just been found in the nuns' toilet. We were dismissed for now and directed to be in study hall in twenty minutes at which time he fully expected the guilty parties to come forward at that time. Then he and the senior prefects dashed off to retrieve the missing pants and clothe the undressed.

The next twenty minutes were bewildering and exhilarating. Most found the episode extremely funny; some were plain happy to have missed mass, many wondered what the punishment should be, and nobody could figure out who the villains were. There was consensus that the skit was one of the best staged ever. The six of us hurriedly held a conclave. We were certain that any sense of humour would be forgotten once universal retribution was applied and the longer we held out, the more severe the consequences. Most importantly, boarding schools have a code of honour and accepting responsibility is very high on that list. We decided not to prolong the suspense, better to confess now and accept our fate.

When we reconvened in the study hall, we had to endure a withering condemnation from the dean. Some laughed which provoked further chastisement. Then he got to the code of honour. Why should all suffer for the sins of a few? Be accountable. Be a man. With that cue, we stood up to face our punishment. We each received six of the leather strap across our palms and wrists on both hands in front of the assembled and we lost the weekly television night and movie night for the rest of the term. For the next two months we sat in the study hall for three hours every Saturday and Sunday night and wrote essays on Hannibal crossing the alps or some such nonsense.

## CHAPTER 12

# KEEP AN OPEN MIND

P arkinson's by its very nature ages you fifteen or twenty years. You walk slower, speak softer. You have to deal with the infirmity of old age well before it's your turn. End of life thoughts flood your consciousness. All of that is natural, but at fifty-five, come on! Now at sixty-one, I sometimes wonder if I will make it to sixty-four, a metric that has some significance to me: the age my father was when he died.

The worst phase of my Parkinson's experience was lurking just around the corner. I had been having cramps in my toes and arches for some time when suddenly they travelled up my body and attacked me above the shoulders. I had cramps from the tiny muscles of my eyelids to the large muscles of my neck. The neck cramps were the most bothersome. The contractions forced my chin to reach for my chest, compressing my neck. Usually, the tightening was hard and to the left. The frightening aspect was the serious restriction on my breathing. It was often scary and always required someone to fight against the contraction and force my neck upright to open up the airway.

I couldn't be alone, particularly in the morning. It required us to be innovative. Patty can see our bedroom window if she sits facing that direction in the kitchen. I stayed in bed as long as I could, partially to allow her to eat and partially to prolong the honeymoon period. The cramping didn't begin until I was fully awake. Dozing delayed the onset. We had a remote-controlled blind on the window facing the kitchen, and we used that as a signal. Just before I fully woke up, I pressed the remote control to raise the window blinds. This alerted Patty that the games were about to begin. The speed of the attacks surprised me every time.

I immediately took my morning 250mg of Sinemet and had to survive until the medicine was sufficiently absorbed by my system to appease the cramping gods. Then Patty got to work manipulating my neck, trying desperately to fight the contraction. It took all her might to combat the seemingly endless assault. The pressure of the tightening was impressive; the muscles felt like aged concrete. Each morning I had to endure considerable discomfort until the Sinemet began to work. It was a battle we could not win. Our aim was to ensure I could breathe.

Once, in the early days of my neck cramps, Patty was struggling to make an impact on the muscle spasms. We were desperate for relief. I had already taken my morning dose of Sinemet with no effect. We were on the verge of calling 911, but we decided to call Suzanne Woody, my massage therapist. Suzanne has gone out of her way to provide me with relief over the last fourteen years. She has learned new techniques on the off chance they would be helpful to me.

She answered her phone and happily agreed to come by the house. She has powerful hands, and we hoped that she could ease the contractions and ideally demonstrate some method that we could replicate each morning. I would have engaged her every morning to work on my neck; she could have moved in.

Patty answered the door and showed her into the living room where I was slouched in a chair with a large heating pad around my taut neck. My head was poking forward like a giant Galapagos turtle, quizzically and at a crooked angle. Come to think of it, my neck was as tight as that turtle's shell. I could not look up to greet her. I had previously forewarned her that I may call some morning, so she was somewhat prepared. Her reaction was still one of shock, but she immediately sprang into action.

I muttered something about lying down, but she instructed, 'Stay right where you are, and I'll work from behind you.'

She moved behind the chair and immediately dug into the tissue. 'Wow, this is really tight.'

Patty said, 'It's been this way for almost thirty minutes now.'

The therapist announced a change of tactic. 'Perhaps if I ease the shoulders and trapezoids, we will get the neck to release.'

She continued to work the upper back areas, but my neck would not capitulate. It became more stubborn to spite her best efforts.

Noticing the increased intensity of my neck cramping she directed me, 'Try to get on the ground. I'll have more leverage if I can get above you.'

Patty and the therapist helped me onto all fours on the ground. She positioned herself above me and used her leverage to attack the source of the cramping. She declared, 'This is like nothing I have seen before.'

Eventually, relief appeared on the horizon. All three of us sat there, equally puzzled. I wondered how much of this I could tolerate. Patty wondered if there was an end in sight. Suzanne wondered what she had just seen.

I'm sure Suzanne helped, but honestly this disease seems to have a mind of its own and for some reason that morning, it chose to make a point by hanging around for over an hour. Apparently, there was little we could do but ride it out and do whatever was necessary to ensure my breathing wasn't obstructed.

This was to be the morning ritual for the next few years; a ritual that lasted for up to forty minutes each and every morning. All the torque on my neck meant it was constantly out of alignment and required three weekly chiropractor visits to adjust and reduce residual pain. I had the good fortune to run into a great doctor whose adjustment procedures rely more on good technique than force – it is your neck and spine after all. My wobbly walking has severely thrown my sacrum out of alignment, and it also needs constant manipulation. Needless to say, I have kept Dr Bennett busy for quite a while now.

Many mornings, other muscle groups got a piece of the action. I frequently had cramps in my calves, quadriceps, hamstrings and even stomach muscles, but none were as scary as the neck cramps, which continued to force me to my hands and knees. I rarely had cramps during the day, once or twice a week only and always when my medicine was at its lowest, an Off Period. It seemed wholly appropriate to increase my daily dosage in an attempt to reduce the effect of the Off Periods and the likelihood of unwelcome cramps during the day.

I was now on 1,500mg of Sinemet daily. This level seemed high and was indicative of how much my condition had deteriorated. I was dosing six times a day, which meant I now had to contend with seven Off Periods each day.

The side effects of this quantity of Sinemet were visible for all to see. As a result, I didn't venture out much. Exceptions were made, but very infrequently. One exception was the Southwest Conference Hall of Fame induction held during a Monday Touchdown Club luncheon in a convention hall in Little Rock.

The Southwest Conference was a highly competitive sports conference that broke up in 1995. The University of Arkansas' departure for the Southeastern Conference three years earlier was likely the catalyst for the breakup. The conference comprised eight Texas Universities and the University of Arkansas. The SWC Hall is part of the Texas Sports Hall of Honor, and they used a football-fan lunch to induct eight former Arkansas sports people. I was included in the chosen ones.

John McDonnell and I had inducted Niall into the previous year's class informally at his home before he died. Naturally, I felt the symmetry of us both coming from the same little town in Ireland had to be recognised. So, I decided that I would risk being a sideshow and attend. I noticed that everyone, especially the organisers, were extremely attentive to me. I was seated close to the dais so that I didn't have to walk too far. A fellow inductee was asked to monitor me while I navigated to the podium.

I made sure I was well medicated and assumed the tremors were under control. I hadn't accounted for the side effects of too much medicine though – the dreaded dyskinesias. I was swaying from side to side like the pendulum of a clock.

The group being inducted included the former women's track coach, Bev Rouse and a former training partner and seven-time NCAA Champion, Joe Falcon. Our coach, John McDonnell, already an inductee, was in the audience. After lunch, the president of the Texas Hall of Honor rose and made his remarks to the over six hundred attendees and welcomed the inductees into the hall.

We were called individually to the dais to receive a memento of our induction and make a few remarks. When it was my turn to approach the microphone, it was all I could do to stand, never mind get to the podium. My minder gave me an arm to lean on, and I traversed what felt like a giant crevasse. The distance was all of six feet. I felt unsteady and a bit rickety. To the audience it must have felt like watching the balance beam in gymnastics, fearing the gymnast will fall off at any moment.

My head was nodding in an up and down motion like a sewing machine. I was in dreadful shape. I guess I had become so accustomed to all the accoutrements of the disease that I didn't realise what a distraction I had become. The gradual nature of the disease progression fools you. After all, you don't wake up in the morning in horrible condition. It's a bit like a glacier; slow moving, but it's coming.

Afterwards, as I chatted with attendees, I kept hearing the same refrain. 'You're so brave.' I don't feel especially brave, so the comment perplexed me.

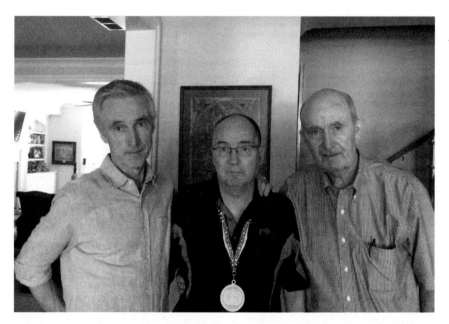

6 September 2015. With John McDonnell, awarding Niall O'Shaughnessy his Southwest Conference Hall of Fame medal.

I mentioned my consternation to a friend a few days later over the phone. He relayed that I looked fine, but added, 'I'm used to it. I see you all the time.'

I responded, 'What does "fine" mean?'

'You didn't look any different than normal.'

'Tell me what "normal" is to you.'

'Normal is ... look, we all know you have Parkinson's. So, whatever that entails.'

'Is it that bad?'

'It's fine.'

'That word again,' I said sarcastically.

We were both a little flustered by now and he could sense it. He offered the following as a truce, 'You ought to see for yourself. The event was streamed. It's probably up on the web by now.'

'Do you know where it was streamed?'

'Surely on the Touchdown Club's Facebook page. I'll find out and get back to you.'

I could think of nothing more important that he could be doing at this juncture. Why was it taking so long to get the name of a streaming site? Of course, he was gainfully employed and was probably in a meeting. A couple of hours later, I received an email with the link to a YouTube video. He warned that it was over two hours long, but I should be on toward the end.

I immediately clicked on the link and found the induction ceremony. I tugged at the tiny red circle on the thin red line at the bottom of the screen multiple times until I found the inductee before me and let it play. I was dismayed at what the next three or four minutes revealed. When my name was called, I received warm applause, but as I pushed back from the table and gingerly made my way to the podium, with assistance, the crowd quietened. Clearly, there was sympathy for my plight or curiosity about what would happen next. Thankfully, I didn't give the audience cause to gasp. I imagine they were juxtaposing the former athlete's prowess against the current model. Athletes should have good genes and should age better than most. Here was the opposite of that perception. Here was a supposed fifty-seven-year-old who seemed more like a seventy-seven-year-old.

I realised then what had prompted the 'bravery' comments. Attendees thought I was courageous to have presented myself in public in that state, to risk scrutiny, to expose my true condition, to perhaps fall. After watching the playbacks, I realised that my shroud of optimism didn't have sufficient fabric; it was threadbare. Seeing the unadulterated response of strangers was elucidating.

My brother, Brendan, who has been firmly in my corner throughout this ordeal, cautioned me to not concern myself with public opinion.

'There are people who will love you no matter what condition you're in and there are others.'

He reminded me how our mother always wanted to leave the best impression possible, too, saying, 'You're too concerned about what others think. Remember how determined Mom was that you arrive in the States in a suit?'

Brendan was already laughing as he began to recount the story.

\* \* \*

The decision to go to the USA was easy for me. My mom wasn't quite so sure, but she understood I wanted to elevate my performances and with reluctance signed the Letter of Intent. Once she was on board, she was totally supportive. As my brother recounted, she was determined that I put my best foot forward, and how better to create a good first impression than to dress nicely? A trip was arranged to McGovern's, a men's clothing shop on William Street in Limerick City. My mother had business dress in mind. I was vaguely aware of how hot it was in the States, and a three-piece wool suit didn't seem appropriate for August.

'You do know it's hot over there?' I protested.

'I realise that,' she said.

'When have you ever been in hot weather?' I enquired.

My mother had lived and worked as a midwife in London in the late forties and fifties, so she said, 'It gets hot in London, and I was on a pilgrimage to Lourdes in Southern France once. It was hot there. Besides, you'll be inside most of the way there,' she added dismissively.

'You want me to wear a suit *flying* there?'

'Francis, you must make a good first impression,' she remonstrated. 'This one would look good on you,' she added, handing me a brown pin-striped number to try on.

I stepped into the dressing room and tried to tug the flimsy curtain shut, but it wasn't broad enough. As soon as I secured one end appropriately, a large gap appeared at the other end. My mother became impatient at my furtive attempts at privacy and urged me to speed things along.

'Francis, nobody's looking. Hurry it up.'

I settled on a centre positioning and managed to get into the suit in the tiny dressing room, which was no bigger than a travel trailer shower. I slid the curtain back and put on the waistcoat as my mother held the jacket for me to put my arms through. She loved it, and I became the proud owner of one brown, woollen pin-striped three-piece suit, once alterations were complete of course.

The morning of my departure for the States I was dressed early. It was late August 1978. In those days, the airport was a big deal. You could have a nice meal and watch the planes take off and land from the observation deck. Many families celebrated big occasions at that restaurant. Indeed, my parents had taken all of us to Shannon Airport for my twin sisters' First Communion a few years earlier. People dressed up then, unlike today's travellers who dress as if they are going to a slumber party or returning from the neighbourhood pool.

Many neighbours and friends had come by to wish me *bon voyage* in the previous few days, so this morning, the visitors were the people I'd miss most: our next-door neighbours, a few close friends and my girlfriend of two years who played a major role in my success as a young athlete and my personal growth. She was an amazing person, and I'm sure she still is. It was a tearful departure, but we promised to write. A promise that she kept, but I didn't do so well at. I did write, but only a few times. I came across a picture she sent me recently. In it she was taking up the gifts during the papal mass in Limerick in front of a million people.

When we got to the airport we met my travel companion, Roddy Gaynor from Sligo. Roddy was entering his second year at the University of Arkansas and had arranged our travel. Our itinerary from Shannon had two stops, one in Gatwick and the other in Dallas, Texas.

Roddy's mother remarked, 'Frank is dressed well.'

'Thank you,' my mother responded as she smiled broadly.

Roddy leaned in and added, 'You know how hot it is over there? You'll fry in that suit.'

'I'll be alright,' I insisted.

We said our goodbyes. It wasn't easy, especially for our parents. We had the excitement of travel, new experiences and school to distract us, while our parents were left to merely worry. I thought about how I felt when I was dropped off at boarding school six years earlier. I was doing the leaving this time. I turned to give my mother a final wave. I could see the tears welling up in her eyes. We both knew at that instant that I likely wasn't coming back.

We landed at Gatwick, and as we taxied to the gate, Roddy explained that we were on standby tickets, and we had to dash to the gate to get our names on the standby list. If there were available seats through either no shows or cancellations, they would be assigned according to the list. We dashed through the terminal to the gate, one fellow in jeans, the other in a suit. We got our names on the list, but we were far from the top.

The ground staff began the boarding process. We would find out after all the ticketed passengers embarked if we would get a seat. We didn't make the flight. We would have to try again tomorrow. We didn't have a credit card between us and decided to spend the night in the airport. We found a relatively quiet area in the giant airport to whittle away the remainder of the day. Our bags were somewhere in the bowels of the airport and beyond our reach. I folded the jacket and waistcoat and draped them over the chair. As I scrunched and levered myself into awkward sleeping positions throughout the night, I did my best to not crease my suit trousers and preserve their crisp lines. When we pulled ourselves together the following morning, I quickly realised I had not been successful. How unsuccessful would require a full-length mirror, which fortunately I didn't have access to.

We immediately got our names on that day's standby list, number one and number two. We spent some of our cash on a full English breakfast at Roddy's insistence. He assured me that I would miss Irish bacon and sausage as much as anything. We again had to wait until the gate was practically closed to determine if our luck had changed, and it had. We had seats on the noon British Airways flight. We were not seated together. I was in the smoking area. So not only would my suit be wrinkled, but it would now reek of smoke. I took the jacket and vest off and placed them in the overhead bin in a futile attempt to protect them from the toxic fumes that were piercing my nostrils.

Eight hours later we landed at DFW International Airport, one of the busiest airports in the world. As we taxied to the gate, I could feel the heat permeating the metal fuselage. It must be steaming hot outside. I grabbed piece one and two of my suit and reluctantly pulled them on. Fellow passengers looked at me in bewilderment as we made our way to the stairs to disembark. There were no gate ramps in those days and a motorised stairs was driven into place. When I poked my head out the door it felt like I had stuck it into a pizza oven. The air was surprisingly dense and heavy and momentarily forced me to hesitate. We had to walk about a hundred metres to the terminal, and I felt every metre. The skin on my face felt like it was broiling. I discovered that brown absorbs heat, and that wool absorbs sweat. Then I encountered the miracle of air conditioning for the first time. As much awe as I felt toward the oppressive heat, I had equal wonderment for air conditioning.

Roddy, who was already inside, remarked, 'Told you it was hot.'

'You never said it was *this* hot.'

'Well, I told you it was too hot for that suit, didn't I?' he retorted.

'What should I do?'

'Change out of it,' he replied.

After we cleared customs, I retrieved some weather-appropriate clothes from my bag and squeezed my suit into the ensuing space created. I had stressed over its condition for the last few days and followed my mother's care instructions. Now at the last barrier, I had discarded it, and much to my mother's chagrin, I would fail to create that first impression she so wanted. After more than thirty-six hours of being over-dressed I arrived under-dressed, looking like someone headed to the neighbourhood pool. If only there was a pool.

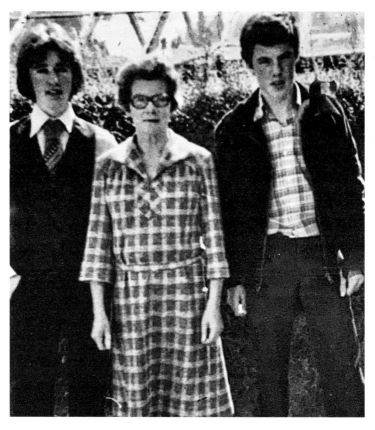

21 August 1978. Dressed for my flight to America with my brother and our neighbour, Evelyn Walsh.

\* \* \*

With Parkinson's there is a real likelihood that you will create a poor first impression. The villain in this act is a common Parkinson's trait that I call 'sour face'. You look like you have a constant scowl on your face, and you appear to be the grumpiest person in the room. An expression of dissatisfaction is stamped on your face with permanent ink. People who don't know all the tentacles of the disease assume you're in a foul mood or upset with them.

There's also 'gawking face'. This is an unintelligent look, characterised by a wide-open mouth and a distant gaze. It may seem you are leering at someone, but really you are a couple of galaxies away.

I found myself saying 'Could you just smile?' as I watched the replay at the Hall of Fame induction.

That public appearance was the watershed moment in my acceptance of the gravity of my situation. The waters parted and it was clear that adjustments had to be made. There were immediate changes I could make and there were more deliberate drastic moves.

My walking had become so unreliable and the risk of falling so great that I had to address it. I knew there was an urgent need for a remedy. I had fallen a couple of times and landed on the pointy edge of both my elbow and hip. Everyone knows nothing good comes from breaking a hip.

Sometimes my legs became entangled and cause me to trip. Alternatively, the toe of my shoe dragged on the floor and the shock threw me off balance. To compound matters, my balance wass seriously compromised. A wheelchair was the obvious solution. I wanted one with a motor – lightweight, fast, with a tight-turning radius. I settled on one called a Zinger. It is steered by pulling or pushing on two handles by the sides so it will turn in very tight spaces and even has a reverse gear with the annoying beeping sound like an earth moving machine.

Getting around the house became much easier, and more importantly, safer. Although it became part of my every day, I can't say I have adjusted fully to a wheelchair mobile life. On days I felt reasonably confident, I dispensed with the chair.

I also decided to avail of disabled parking. Badges are easy enough to acquire but their usage requires a certain amount of callousness. People covet the proximity and wonder what you did to acquire such a pass. I am convinced that onlookers are watching those first few steps to evaluate whether you are badge-worthy. Unfortunately, for me, I quickly dispel the presumed ruse with my first lunge toward the store entrance. I try to not overuse the privilege. I won't sit in the car in a disabled spot waiting for someone who wants to be dropped off close. On the odd occasion when I can sort of walk, I will park in the burbs.

I vowed to keep active. I have the luxury of having a home gym set-up that includes a treadmill. I often get on the treadmill and within a half mile I can no longer walk, but I use my arms to balance myself on the side railings and take some weight off my legs. This allows me to continue on for another mile. It's not exactly walking, but you have to keep moving somehow. On a good day I walk, or quasi-walk, two miles. For some reason I struggle to walk on an incline and to a lesser degree on a decline, so I generally stay on the flat indoor surface. I find that the more I push myself, the more I can accomplish.

Ultimately, I knew these moves were only a balm and I would have to undergo a more invasive solution.

## CHAPTER 13

# TAKE A WALK IN THEIR SHOES

**B**efore you achieve you have to imagine. Our dreams are pure and uncontaminated, and have yet to be subjected to life's tumble dryer of doubt, insecurities and lethargy. Most childhood dreams are destroyed by doubters and naysayers or are un-nurtured by family or friends. I have been fortunate to have mentors or sponsors at every juncture in life who reinforced my goals and aspirations. Many kind people gave invaluable advice, dispelled doubts and invested time in me. This was especially true at St Munchin's and at my clubs, Limerick Athletic Club and Emerald Athletic Club. Fortunately, I have mostly been around positive people or perhaps I innately knew to filter those energy sappers from my life.

It was when I crossed the pond that I figured out how much effort was required to make your dreams come true. Like most Irish, I had a strong attachment to the USA. A huge percentage of my ancestors have emigrated to the States over the years. Not so much my generation; I am one of two in my generation to leave Ireland. Strange, then, that two of my grandparents emigrated to the USA around the end of the nineteenth century. My father's father, with whom I share a first name, worked as a silver miner in Leadville, Colorado in the 1870s. He could have died like so many did in a mining accident or of some pesky disease that frequently engulfs mining towns. It has been estimated that over 1,400 Irish lost their lives in the Leadville area during that era. Luckily, he survived the perils of living in a frontier town and made it back to Flagmount in County Clare. As fortuitous as we are that he survived in that environment, we are equally fortunate that he came home. Not many did in the late 1800s.

I was doubly blessed by the emigration gods. My mother's mother, Nellie Sullivan, emigrated to the USA when she was younger and also returned. What are the odds that both grandparents would come back home? My grandmother moved to Boston in the early 1900s where she worked as a nanny. It couldn't have been loneliness that spurred her to return; she had nine siblings in the Boston area. Apparently, she went home to help her aging father. I imagine she and her siblings drew straws, and she had the shortest. Either way, she was back in Kenmare, County Kerry and married a year later.

She was a lovely lady and very devout. She would kneel on the hard wood floor and pray for hours. She prayed for everyone: family, friends, neighbours, people she read about in the church bulletin or her *Messenger* booklet. Many times, I saw her kneeling on the hallway floor next to the radiator to keep warm. I know because she lived with us. She moved in after I was born and never left. For all intents and purposes, I had three parents. She even outlived my father. Her simple life and her extreme devotion were an inspiration to me.

In her later years, she lived in a nursing home close to Shannon Airport. My mother told me that every time she heard a Boeing 747 fly overhead, she would say that was her grandson coming home. Fortunately, I never missed a Christmas in Ireland and was at home every summer until Parkinson's got its nasty claws in me.

I would stop by to see her on my way back to America. She would cry when I left, and it always pulled at my heartstrings. She'd say, 'Francis, you will write to me and tell me all about your life in America, won't you?'

'I will, Granny.'

'And let me know how that actor is doing as president,' she added for a few years.

I think she was jealous that I got to live in America.

Since arriving in the USA in the fall of 1978, I have always lived in Arkansas and the state has been good to me. Two institutions in particular have played a huge part in my life: the University of Arkansas where I was coached for seventeen years by the incomparable John McDonnell and Alltel Wireless where I was hired by the inspirational Scott Ford and where I was employed in one fashion or another for another spell of fourteen years.

The year after I honoured that promise to my father by comprehensively winning the All-Ireland Schools Intermediate 1,500m, I finished fifth in the senior version in a time that was ten seconds slower. I did manage two victories in the FISEC games in Linz, Austria. Shortly after my return from those two victories on the continent, the All-Ireland Junior Championships were held at my home track. Most significantly, Coach McDonnell, who was recruiting me to run for the University of Arkansas, was in attendance.

In those days, receiving a scholarship to represent a US university was the crowning achievement for an Irish schoolboy athlete. If I were to hazard a guess, I would say that close to a thousand Irish teenagers have accepted athletics scholarships since John Joe Barry first left Irish shores for Villanova University in 1950. Many of those scholarship recipients have enjoyed tremendous success both athletically and professionally. I hope all made good use of the opportunity presented to them.

Many young athletes forgo the US collegiate path these days. Facilities in Ireland are much better than they were; coaching has improved and there are many more opportunities in Ireland now than there were in our era. There were two tartan tracks in the republic when I left in 1978 and both were in Dublin. We had no choice; we had to leave to improve, and I feel that sacrifice strengthened us.

One of my competitors that afternoon in Limerick was Dave Taylor. I didn't know Dave. He was a year older than I, and we competed in different age brackets. He turned out to be a formidable athlete who got the better of me that day in Limerick and did so with some frequency over the next few years. John had written in his recruiting letter that he only had one scholarship available for mid-distance runners, and I was his first choice. Well, now he had a predicament. Does he change horses before the beginning of the NCAA season? I had not accepted his offer, so John was free to choose another athlete.

The Limerick track was surrounded entirely by a grass bowl. Spectators brought blankets and sat or lay on the grass, all spread out in a bunch. The bowl was also tall enough to offer magnificent surveillance points. As I sat high up on the berm lamenting my loss with my school coach, we spotted John and the newly crowned Irish junior champion immersed in serious conversation.

My coach said, 'Isn't that the winner of your race talking to the Arkansas coach?'

'I can't really tell. It looks like the colours he was wearing.' I had not met Dave Taylor and could not pick him out in a crowd.

'Wonder what they are discussing?' he said.

'He'd never … would he?'

'You get two guesses, and the first one doesn't count.'

'He did tell me I was his number one choice.'

'You need to go talk to him, and make sure he knows you won in Austria last week.'

'Agreed, I'll do it.'

'Tell him you were tired from the travel,' were his parting words.

I was nervous. John was clearly fascinated with the lanky ex-footballer. He only had one scholarship remaining and must have been persuaded by Dave's dominating performance that day. I wondered for a moment should I ask Dave what they discussed. I had barely spoken to him and that didn't feel appropriate. For all I knew, he might tell me to mind my own business.

I angled up to John sheepishly. His choice would have been a lot simpler had I won that day. He got right to the point. 'I was expecting to see that kick everyone's been talking about. What happened?'

'I guess I was a little tired. I just got back from Austria.'

Then he offered, 'You did look tired out there and you had no answer when the Taylor kid upped the pace. Do you know much about him?'

'No, sir, I've never seen him before, but you know I'm a year younger,' I anxiously responded.

John recognised my anguish and said, 'Don't worry, kid. I want the Taylor lad in addition to you.'

'But I thought there was only one scholarship available?'

John managed to wiggle out of answering that one, but kept his word. The freshman class of distance runners that fall included not only O'Mara from Limerick and now Dave Taylor from Dublin, but a third – Randy

Stephens from Birmingham, Alabama. Not one middle-distance runner on scholarship, but three. So much for, 'I've only got one scholarship for a distance runner.' Both the other freshmen had stellar college careers. Randy won Arkansas's first individual NCAA Indoor title and Dave was twice in the top ten at the cross-country nationals and a 3:54 miler. Randy was my roommate. We immediately bonded over, of all things, the one vinyl record I brought with me from home, 'One more from the road', a live recording of Lynyrd Skynyrd whose best-known track was 'Sweet Home Alabama'.

John coached me for seventeen years and gave me an assistant coach's role after graduation. He encouraged me to pursue an MBA while on the university's payroll and was again supportive of me while I juggled law school and athletics. Working for him was my introduction to servant leadership. He led by example. He did more work than any of his assistants or athletes. He kept it simple and repeatable. I watched him win forty-two national team titles and was inspired at how humble he remained given his enormous success.

During my days as a student at the university, I and a few teammates signed up to play intramural water polo. Now before you are too impressed, I should point out that we played in inner tubes. I, for one, could not tread water with nearly the skill required for real water polo. One day, our pole vaulter brought along another student to augment our team, his cousin, Scott Ford, from Little Rock. The tournament required that we play every team once, and the top two teams met in the final. Scott made a few appearances for us, and we managed to make the final. The final was delayed for one reason or another. Some of us hadn't eaten, so Scott drove to a restaurant and brought everyone back a sandwich. We liked him from the beginning.

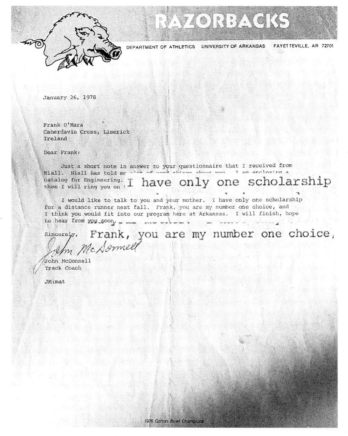

26 January 1978. 'I only have one scholarship' recruiting letter from the University of Arkansas.

I saw Scott at a few university functions during our time in Fayetteville, and he was always engaging. After college, he moved to New York to pursue a career in investment banking. I ran into him once while in New York for a race. We were both shopping in a department store and saw one another as we travelled in opposite directions on facing escalators. After some confusion and hand gesturing over which one of us would stay and which would ride to the other's floor, we greeted each other and spent ten minutes or so catching up. We didn't see each other again for ten years.

In the spring of 1996, despite having achieved the qualifying standard for a fourth Olympics that summer, I retired from professional athletics because of persistent trouble with my left leg and back. I was looking for a job and I was desperate for a meaningful role in an evolving technology industry; nobody knows what development is around the corner, and so everybody learns together. I was thirty-six entering the workforce, and I was used to independence. I had no desire to be supervised by some middle-aged middle manager. I didn't have contacts at technology companies, so the solution had to be to work for myself.

We had two young sons by then, so we put a premium on being close to family. That narrowed the search ring down to Little Rock or Limerick. My vote was Limerick. I heard from my friend, Pat Chesser, that the two McDonalds in my hometown were for sale, and I decided to pursue the possibility of acquiring them. McDonald's franchises at that time were virtually money machines. I could make a great living in my hometown.

First, I needed approval from the McDonald's franchisee people in Chicago. It took a tedious couple of months before I was finally approved as a potential McDonald's franchisee in early December. The next step was to work in an actual store to test my interest. I was scheduled to work five days as a Franchisee in Training in a store in North London. If I could get past this step, I could buy the two stores in Limerick and move home.

My first day at McDonald's was 18 December 1996, a week before Christmas, an especially busy time with shoppers in high gear. I was staying at my agent, Kim McDonald's, apartment in Teddington, London. I suited up in the work clothes I had been sent and pinned on my OJE (On the Job Evaluation) button. I was excited as I drove across London in Kim's Porsche dressed in McDonald's attire, a funny sight no doubt.

The store was so busy the morning flashed by. But after lunch, the day began to drag, and the monotony of my one task became unbearable. How many bags of potatoes can you tip into boiling fat? The other twenty-one employees weren't unpleasant, but they made sure I was confined to the fryer all day. The OJE button only served to remind them that I was being

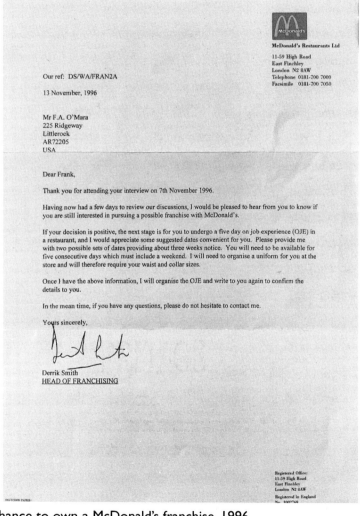

My chance to own a McDonald's franchise, 1996.

groomed for management, or maybe they saw me arrive in that Porsche. I worked twelve hours that day and arrived back at Kim's, exhausted.

On morning two, I woke up and thought, 'What is that awful smell?' It was the lingering odour of fried food, and it was coming from my only uniform. I reluctantly pulled the shirt over my back. It reminded me of not wanting to put a shirt on the morning after a sunburn. The Franchisee in Training programme is designed to separate those who are most suited from those merely interested in financial rewards. It certainly did with me. It took two days to establish that I didn't have the stomach to be a golden archer.

I continued to provide McDonald's with free labour for the agreed five days; and yes, I did wear that same uniform the entire time, but no, I didn't drive the Porsche. I woke earlier and took public transport. Disappointingly, I never even got to work the drive-through window which seemed the pinnacle of achievement. I did work at the griddle and still marvel that a rock-hard hamburger patty, taken out of the freezer and placed directly on the griddle, will cook fully in forty-seven seconds with the upper cooking surface lowered.

Most people I told about that adventure wondered why I completed the five days. It wasn't for fear that my mind would change, but fulfilment of my end of a bargain. Without a doubt, those five days gave me perspective and an understanding of what some have to endure to make a living.

I got back to Little Rock two days before Christmas. I had retired from running over nine months earlier, and I had two children and little income or health insurance. The only money I had made over that period was for TV commentary at the Atlanta Olympics, a role I reprised at the Sydney Olympics, and part time legal work for Kim McDonald International

Management (KIM).

A friend suggested I interview with Scott Ford, who was now the President and COO of Alltel Corporation, a Fortune 500 company, based in Little Rock. Alltel had a wireline and information technology businesses – and a more interesting nascent mobile phone provider business. Scott saw the future in wireless and was building a team to launch a digital wireless network. I, on the other hand, had limited work experience, but I was well educated and a member of the Arkansas Bar.

I did have many interesting life experiences. I had won World Championships with millions watching, and I had greatly disappointed in front of millions too. I knew how to keep going in the face of adversity. Scott likely remembered that I grew up the son of a small-business owner and likely had understood the value of a dollar. He took a chance on a college acquaintance and gave me an opportunity for which I am eternally grateful.

In the first few months of my employment, I struggled with the sudden discipline mandated by a standard forty-hour work week. I was accustomed to total independence and without any acclimatisation, now had less control than Canute had over the tide. I promised myself that I wouldn't pass judgement on my new existence for six months. By that time, I should be more accustomed to the routine. When I finally evaluated my new life, I realised that I loved the place, the people, the industry. I was relieved to have made the transition.

Scott championed my career and gave me endless opportunities to excel. It wasn't always rosy though. A few years into my tenure, there was a particular occasion where Scott had good cause to call me at home at night. I had taken on the role of chief marketing officer and discovered that nobody in that department kept a proper promotional calendar. This calendar should contain all upcoming promotional plans for at least nine months to a year. It often takes that long to update the billing system to include the promotional pricing, to produce appropriate commercials, arrange for phone inventory and much more. When a promotion is not well staged, there often are execution issues which generate calls to our customer service centres and visits to our stores. The next promotional window was 'Back to School' in a couple of months and no coordinated planning had been done.

I did find one comprehensive plan. The director of diversity marketing had developed a 'Back to School' programme for our larger urban markets. It contained all the essential elements. It was a textbook example of proper planning. I decided to highlight her work as an example to the other directors of what was expected. I directed the team to leverage her programme into a back-to-school promotion for the entire country. The programme included a clear backpack and notepad, other school supplies featuring a well-known rap artist and a recording of a new track by that artist. The diversity director had worked for months on her plan, and she had every angle covered. It would be easy to replicate.

Rap music isn't everyone's favourite genre. Most objections stem from the lyrics and the influence of gangs and crime. It would be a hard sell in rural America. I asked to review the lyrics before committing and found them a little objectionable, but tolerable. I gambled and decided to expand the campaign to all markets.

The rapper plan would be live on Monday, and the stores received their shipment of promotional material on Thursday, everything from window clings to inventory.

It turned out that some of the artist's previous work was downright offensive, causing some of our regional management staff to call the boss and complain. Immediately, Scott picked up the phone and called me.

The phone rang at home around 8pm.

'Frank, this is Scott. I'm going to read something to you, and you tell me what you think of it.'

Scott then read me the lyrics of one of the artist's earlier works.

'Well, what do you think of that?'

'Pretty awful,' I agreed.

'Do you know what that is from?' he asked, more annoyed than angry.

'I'm guessing it's from the rapper in our back-to-school promotion,' I sheepishly responded.

'You're right, and I want this nonsense removed from all our stores immediately,' he demanded.

'I reviewed his current material, and it's edgy but acceptable. The stuff you read is old material.'

I had been assured the artist was older and had moved on from his old ways when I asked the diversity director about his earlier work. I had applied the wisdom of Wilde once again. 'Every saint has a past, every sinner has a future.'

'We don't need to be associated with this,' Scott continued.

'Who is complaining, anyway?' I asked.

'A regional sales manager complained.'

I asked, 'Can I give you my side of the story before we pull the promotion?'

I outlined my rationale. I acknowledged that it was a troublesome promotion, but told him I needed our marketing team to properly plan and execute. I added that the diversity marketing director had done all that and more. I wanted to reward her and send a message to the other team members that expectations had been raised.

'Trust me on this. The harm we would cause by pulling the programme is far greater than any damage the campaign could even conceivably create.' I added, 'We haven't received a customer complaint, have we?'

'Okay, let it run, but let's watch it closely.' And with that remonstrance, Scott conceded.

If he had pulled the plug on the maligned campaign, it may well have been the finish of my burgeoning marketing career. Certainly, it would have taken ages to reestablish my leadership credentials within the marketing and sales departments. Scott was by nature an enlightened leader. He was prepared to hand over responsibility and trusted you to get it done. Great leaders develop others to lead, and he allowed me to set the tone in sales and marketing.

That was as rocky as it ever was between us. He didn't agree with the decision, but understood the predicament I was in. I didn't much like my decision either, and I knew that once made, there was no backing down. Needless to say, it was a short-lived promotion, and we were ready for the fall promotion in all markets and for all segments.

Scott made major leadership changes during his tenure, sold the Information Technology branch and spun off the Wireline business. His informed changes and inspiring leadership transformed Alltel into the fifth largest wireless provider in the US with a little less than thirteen million customers and around ten billion dollars in revenue before Alltel was bought by Verizon for 28.1 billion dollars in 2009, when this story begins.

Growing up I could never claim to have been driven by my parents to be a success. Indeed, a good civil service job would have pleased my mother just fine. I think she was fearful of overreaching, a little bit of Catholic anxiety that bad things are only waiting to happen. Often, she would caution against a particular objective as if it was beyond our reach, something reserved for others of a higher station in life. Fortunately, we had some of our father's bottomless optimism. In fairness to my mother, she did exhort us to always give our full effort, to always complete a task.

It was when I got to Arkansas that I was encouraged by John McDonnell to extend my horizons further, to establish real goals and to hold myself accountable. Scott gave me platforms to apply those raw skills in the business world, he supported me through sharp learning curves. Both understood that to be a great leader you could not rely solely on your formal authority. You need an emotional attachment to your team.

In extreme environments or under unusual duress, formal authority is often challenged, and an emotional leader emerges from the group. A team needs a leader who creates optimism and fosters camaraderie. This role was thrust upon Shackleton on his 1901 *Discovery* voyage to the Antarctic. Captain Robert Scott of the Royal Navy was the senior officer in command of the ship, but, when everything turned bleak, he holed up in his cabin. The men gravitated toward Shackleton who lifted their spirits with his steadfastness. This undermined Scott's effectiveness. Scott eventually sent Shackleton home when a ship appeared to restock the *Discovery*.

John and Scott avoided this dilemma. They created loyalty by recognising the work of others, supporting them and putting in an honest shift themselves. Ultimately, we would have run through a wall for either.

## CHAPTER 14

# STAY CURRENT, STAY RELEVANT

I remember watching the NBC broadcast of the Olympic cycling road race in 2008. One of the US riders was Taylor Phinney whose mother and father were both Olympians. Taylor's father, Davis, was diagnosed with Parkinson's at forty and the disease had developed sufficiently to merit Deep Brain Stimulation (DBS). During the Olympic bike race telecast the network featured his DBS surgery as part of a biographical piece on Taylor. Davis had some sort of restraining device on his head, and he was secured to the table. There was a doctor standing behind him apparently drilling into his skull and, shockingly, he was wide awake and conversing with the surgeons. I recollect thinking how barbaric the procedure looked and how brave he was to endure such an ordeal. 'How bad must this disease be to merit such a procedure?' The piece ended and I thought, 'Thank God, I'll never be in that predicament.' This was six months before my first symptom. I had an innate, organic fear of DBS.

Yet here I was discussing the same possibility with my doctors. I had exhausted all the drug protocol possibilities. The only other option was to throw my hands in the air and accept my fate. It was a simple case of desperate measures for desperate times. I wanted a shot at reclaiming some portion of my previous life.

I completely trusted both doctors' judgement and heeded their advice to begin the approval process for deep brain stimulation. Approval is not simply given once sought. The procedure at the Mayo Clinic requires an evaluation by a committee of experts in various neurology specialties. These experts independently examine the candidate and meet periodically to review each case. The committee votes on every applicant's suitability for the procedure. If approved, the candidate is added to the surgical list and awaits a scheduling call. It could take eighteen months to two years to get a slot, so best to declare an interest early.

DBS works on the theory that an electric current introduced to the part of the brain that is generating the faulty signalling will interfere with and prevent those signals from occurring. This forces the brain to find alternate routes for signalling. The process has three stages. The first is a four-to-five-hour surgery during which two dime-sized holes are drilled in the cranium and two leads, each with four electrodes, are implanted deep in the brain. My target area was the Subthalamic Nucleus (STN), a part of the substania nigra.

The second stage, a week later, is a one-to-two-hour surgery to implant a neurostimulator in the chest and then tunnel the wiring beneath the skin of the chest and neck and under the scalp to connect with wiring the leads. The neurotransmitter supplies the electrical pulses that will be delivered via the leads.

During the third stage, another week later, the neurotransmitter is turned on and programmed for the first time. It would have been tested in the second procedure, but this is the first time the movement disorder specialist will strive to optimise settings.

I visited with some local DBS patients, none of whom regretted having had the surgery and all of whom remarked that they had seen noted improvement. I did notice one unpleasant feature of each. The cap that was designed to seal the two holes toward the front of the hairline had left noticeable bumps. I must say they were a little distracting. I resolved to enquire about the finishing touches upon my appointment at Mayo.

My first visit to the Mayo Clinic was to establish a definitive diagnosis. My dalliance with Lyme left a shadow and I had to know for certain if I ever had the disease. Mayo had substantial experience with Lyme given its prevalence in Minnesota. A lumbar puncture was performed to confirm or deny that I had Lyme disease. The result was negative, so if I ever had Lyme disease, it was now gone. I paused for a few moments and rued all the suffering I had needlessly endured and then I decided it was time to move on. It was just like another defeat that had to be processed and learned from. There's no point looking backward. After two days, I left with a definitive diagnosis of Early Onset Idiopathic Parkinson's Disease.

Next step was a full week's screening for deep brain stimulation approval. The first morning was the most worrisome. The first test is essentially a before and after examination. Your condition prior to your first helping of Sinemet that day is compared to your condition after. At that time, I was heavily reliant on Sinemet, taking over 1,800mg per day. I was deep in the neck-cramping phase and forewarned the medical staff that it could be ugly and even problematic. They assured me I could take my Sinemet shortly after arrival because of the medicine's absorption period. This would give them roughly thirty minutes to complete before the Sinemet kicked in.

We stayed in a hotel immediately across the street from the Clinic's main entrance. The evening before I could barely walk that short distance, so we arranged for a wheelchair. The next morning, I woke to the usual cramping sequence. My legs were as stiff as metal rods, and my chin was attached to my chest. I wore a heating pad around my neck like a collar to counter the contractions. I unceremoniously slumped into the wheelchair. My left leg was as rigid as a poker and was unapologetically sticking straight out in front of me, rendering navigation quite difficult.

My appointment was the earliest available, but it overlapped with staff arriving for work and patients for the day's first appointments. It was hustle and bustle with people juggling coffee mugs and keys and wallets. All the traffic was merging at the elevators, a morning rush hour crowd of pedestrians. By now, my neck was severely contracted, and my leg was rigid and acting like a battering ram. Navigation wasn't simple for Patty. I tried to ignore all the people, some doing their best to assist, some doing their best to avert their eyes while Patty tried to thank everyone. By the time we arrived on the appointed floor after stops at every floor on the way, the staff were waiting and whisked us into a room instantly.

The purpose of the first inspection was to establish my baseline Uniform Parkinson's Disease Rating Scale (UPDRS) score. The rating scale is designed to gauge the disease's progression and includes both motor and non-motor symptoms. The tests are simple but illustrative, and each test is scored zero to four, with four being the worst. There is no minimum score required for surgery. Rather, you are expected to show improvement between both scores. Responsiveness to Sinemet is the leading indicator of a positive reaction to deep brain stimulation.

At that moment, these tests separated me from my life-giving Sinemet. Fortunately, the nurse performing the tests was conscious of my plight and was as speedy as she could be. I had been scored on the UPDRS scale before, but not understanding its purpose, I had no interest in my scores. Moreover, the tests seemed so elementary and the scoring so subjective. Now, the same tests were standing between me and surgery.

I performed poorly on the prescribed tests. My neck was so cramped that I could not raise my eyes to look at the nurse, nor could I nod my head to affirm any of her directives. I could only mutter and hope Patty could translate. I believe the first test was to hold my hands out straight and make fists as fast as I could. I barely managed to raise my arms, and the fist making was slow and minute. The second test was tapping the index finger and thumb together as hard as possible. I could just about bring the two digits together. It took all my determination to separate them.

There was a clear contrast between these tests and the first tests administered to me by Dr Archer ten years earlier. Back then, I felt I had distinguished myself. It took a well-trained eye to see otherwise. This time I would need to have been a hundred per cent delusional to find any competency. A side-by-side video of both would have been sobering. I looked at Patty despairingly. She knew what I was thinking, and she nodded.

On we went. The nurse was exceedingly patient and understanding as I laboured from one test to another. The whole time, Patty massaged my neck and did her best to translate. I was in almost total lockdown trying to survive until I could take my first Sinemet of the day. I was still sitting in the wheelchair with my left leg as stiff as a flagpole protruding to the middle of the room. I couldn't lower it for love nor money. Halfway through the 'before testing' the nurse suggested that I take the medication. With the end in sight, we powered through the remainder. She then left the room and directed us to alert her once the Sinemet had fully kicked in. That took the bones of another twenty minutes, and Patty notified her that I was no longer a part of *The Walking Dead* cast.

I greeted the nurse when she arrived back in the room as if it was the first time we had met. I couldn't look up at her the previous time. She then took me through the same battery of tests we had just completed, but for this attempt there was some petrol in the tank. I fared much better the second offering. I could open and close my fists competently, tap my feet well and was understandable.

I didn't know what I had scored on the earlier 'off' test portion, but I knew the second 'on' score was much lower. I was also aware that the paramount concern for approval was the candidate's responsiveness to Sinemet. There would be another three days' worth of appointments and countless evaluations, but this one was critical. It turned out my 'before' score was fifty-one, which was characterised as 'severe', and my reaction to the medication was as desired. My 'after' score was eleven.

There were evaluations of speech and gait, but the second most challenging evaluation was cognitive testing. Dementia has a high occurrence rate among those afflicted with Parkinson's, and unfortunately anyone who illustrates even the early signs of this horrible condition is not a DBS candidate. Therefore, the screening is rigorous. It involves your ability to recall earlier words and perform tasks while being constantly confused and distracted with new words and challenges. It's specifically designed to test your memory when you are confused and tired. The practitioner changed the rules and the format constantly in varying attempts to rattle and frustrate. The whole affair was comparable to a police interrogation where the suspect tires of the scrutiny, throws her hands in the air and says, 'Okay, you got me. Just make this stop.'

After thirteen appointments in three days, we were done. The staff at the

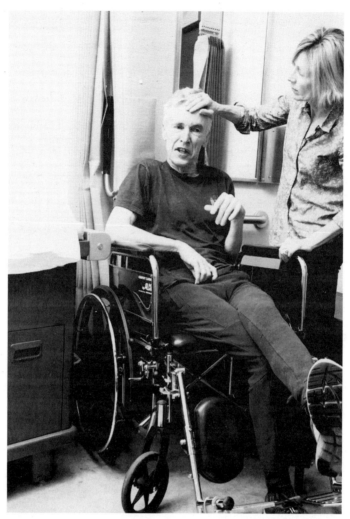

17 May 2018. Before my first Sinemet at the Pre-DBS evaluation.

clinic were extraordinarily attentive and caring, from the neurologists to nurses to porters, everyone was pulling in concert. We felt especially good when the neurosurgeon who would perform the surgery declared that my Parkinson's symptoms were ideal targets for DBS.

The recurring theme among the evaluations was I had extreme dyskinesia, was very rigid and had severe cramping, all of which are in the target zone for DBS. We headed home to consider the prospect of the surgery.

The moment I set foot at home, I began to worry about the trauma of the surgery. Patty was anxious for a call saying I had been approved and was on the surgery schedule. I was in no hurry for the phone to ring. I put up a charade of impatience waiting for the call. In reality, I was buying time.

Patty didn't understand my reticence, but she kept encouraging me. Through it all, she had been there for me, and she was there now as I went through this period of doubt.

Then I got a call from a former teammate, Harold Smith, who is a neurosurgeon and has performed some three hundred of this exact surgery. He turned out to be a crutch I could lean on. He was a source of great encouragement throughout the waiting period. He reinforced that I was a perfect patient for DBS and would be foolish not to stay the course.

We spoke regularly. I remember one conversation, when he reassured me, 'Listening to you describe your symptoms, I know this surgery will give you tremendous relief.'

'So, you have seen patients with a similar presentation make an improvement?' I asked.

'Dramatic, and your presentation makes you an ideal candidate for this procedure,' he said.

'That's great, Harold!'

'I'll tell you another thing. I'm going to be at that surgery with you. Let me know when you get the date, and I'll clear the decks.'

'Harold, that's beyond considerate of you.'

'Meanwhile, let's check in periodically. Okay?'

Harold mentioned in a subsequent conversation that he had just begun using a new technology by a medical manufacturer called Abbot. I knew a thing or two about technology from my days in the wireless world. Namely, I knew technology can change quickly. The current state of the art can be yesterday's news in an instant. Technology tends to make step function changes, stay relatively quiet for a few years then another improvement. I had to be certain I didn't put soon-to-be-outdated equipment in my brain. You have one shot to get the leads right.

The more I learned about Neuromodulation, the more I realised the industry was on the precipice of major growth and change. For many years, lead technology had remained constant. Each lead contained four separate omni-directional electrodes emitting current in a 360-degree pattern. If the lead is placed too close to the edge of the target area, an electrode can unwittingly stimulate a neighbouring area, causing any number of unwanted consequences including compromised balance or slurred speech. Your only option is to turn that electrode off completely. Wouldn't the lead have more utility if it had the capacity to turn off a portion of a specific electrode? Particularly when the target area is the size of a grain of rice. Harold was patient and explained all the intricacies to me. He had converted to multi-directional leads in his surgeries and was pleased with the outcomes. He shared articles to read, and I was convinced that multi-directional was the way to go.

The call came; I was approved for deep brain stimulation surgery. We both were elated and nervous. I still didn't have a date. That would come in the near future call from the surgeon. I read the words 'near future' and thought, *This is happening way too fast. Slow down. Let's take stock of the situation for a second.*

I relayed that fear to Patty. 'I don't know if I am ready for this. Do I really have to?'

'Frank, come on now. You know you need this,' she replied.

'But it's brain surgery, and I have to be awake the entire time.' That's correct awake, and alert for the duration.

Patty responded, 'We met the surgeon, and you liked him … right?'

'For sure, he seemed confident.'

'He has done over a thousand of these, and he said he can help you. You're in safe hands.'

I received intermittent calls from the movement-disorder specialists at Mayo. They would be responsible for adjusting the pulse generator after surgery. They also would play a critical role during the procedure, administering tests to confirm the leads were appropriately placed during surgery.

I mentioned to them my interest in multi-directional technology. Each time, they convinced me otherwise. They had valid reasons such as familiarity with the existing implementation process and the fear of unknown outcomes. I couldn't muster the courage to insist.

I called Harold, and he reminded me that with my technology background, I should understand the benefits of being current. This was tested and approved equipment. Above all, he reminded me, 'It's your body and your decision.'

I was braver on the next teleconference. This call was the last before surgery. The caller was going through a checklist of what to expect, what to bring, how long we would be there. Suddenly she said, 'We will be implanting Medtonic equipment.'

Instinctively, I blurted out, 'I'd prefer if we could use the new Abbot leads.'

'I don't know if we have used the Abbot equipment.'

Then the comment that makes many in the medical community cringe.

'I'm doing some research on the web, and I think Abbot gives me the greatest optionality in the future.'

'I'll check with Dr Lee,' she replied.

I was relieved. I had stood my ground and chosen the prickly option. I would be disappointed, but would understand if the answer was negative. Happily, I got a call back saying that Dr Lee had agreed to use the Abbot equipment.

My inability to keep weight on had become worrisome. Severe dyskinesia meant my body was in constant motion. When I sat, my neck craned, and my head nodded. My arms swung uncontrollably when I walked. There were the daily cramping events and tremors. All of this activity required an energy source, and consequently, I had lost a lot of body mass.

I was determined to be in the best possible condition for surgery. I needed to gain weight and strength. Initially, I was prescribed high-calorie milkshakes with the direction to consume five thousand calories a day. I should have read the contents label and seen the protein content. I also should have recalled that protein limits the ability to absorb Sinemet into the blood stream. The general rule of thumb is no protein for two hours before and one hour after dopamine medication.

I just introduced a mountain of additional protein into my diet. The increased protein level meant my Sinemet was less effective even to the extreme of not working at all. These ramifications occurred within twenty-four hours of ingesting the first shake. I did manage to tolerate the undesired response for four or five days to confirm the milkshakes were the problem. Through various other methods I managed to gain five pounds. I augmented my diet with strength work. I set a goal to bench press my body weight prior to surgery, and I managed 130 pounds, which put me over the hurdle. I was as ready as I would be.

## CHAPTER 15

# SURROUND YOURSELF WITH POSITIVE PEOPLE

The date chosen for deep brain stimulation was 9 January 2019, which, by sheer coincidence, was ten years to the very day since I had my first apparent symptom while running with friends. The three parts of DBS occurred over a two-week window, and we were advised to spend the entire period in Rochester. We had to be at the clinic two days before the first surgery. There is no paucity of worry-worthy items, but thankfully my good friend, Rick Massey, handled all the travel and logistics, so I could cross that off the list.

My sister, Ann, travelled over from Ireland to accompany us to Rochester. We chose the same hotel directly across the road from the clinic. We were regular visitors by now, and they gave us a roomy corner suite. My other sister, Helen, arrived from Ireland the next day and my son, Jack, was coming for round two. So, we needed living space. A guest of honour was coming all the way from Lubbock, Texas, Dr Harold Smith, who had coached me through this journey and led me to a wise technology selection.

When we arrived in Rochester, snow was falling from a heavy sky. It was everywhere; mounds taller than streetlights lined every roadside. There was so much snow downtown that they had to truck it out to the country. Luckily, there is a very extensive underground shopping and pedestrian system in the downtown area, consisting of a labyrinth of shops and alleyways much like you picture in a Turkish bazaar. Helen arrived in the late afternoon just in time for all of us to get lost in the underground. It was difficult to decipher which stairwell would release us closest to the above ground restaurant where we had reservations. We were like prairie dogs emerging from holes as we tried different exits.

Our first appointment the next day was at the reasonable time of 10:15 with the man I was about to entrust with my life, whatever remained of it, Dr Kendall Lee. To say he made us feel like he was up to the challenge would be the understatement of the year. Confidence oozed from every pore. It wasn't the bothersome or irksome kind in any way. It was the sort born from extensive experience; he had performed this surgery almost a thousand times with great outcomes and no infections. An infection in the brain was a particular worry for me. He squashed any concern and reaffirmed that he believed I was an excellent candidate and would greatly benefit from surgery.

We briefly discussed the Abbot equipment that I had asked for, and he proclaimed it shouldn't be an issue. He added that the Abbot people would be here for the pre-operation meeting. He had also developed his own caps, which prevented the hump effect I had seen in some who had undergone DBS.

He alerted us to look out for a phenomenon called the 'honeymoon period'. I should experience this effect between the two surgeries. In many patients who undergo DBS surgery, the mere fact that the surgeon has placed the lead in the STN, triggers a positive response. Although the neurotransmitter will not be implanted for another week, the patient can feel the sought-after effect. For most, the effect lasts a couple of days. The very fact that you experience a honeymoon effect is a good indicator of a positive response to DBS. The longer and stronger the response, the more encouraged the surgeon is of the outcome.

We left the consultation happy and sure that I was in safe hands.

My sister, Ann, who is a nurse by training, even declared, 'That's the most genuinely confident doctor I have ever met.'

Patty added, 'I think he's confident and not arrogant.'

I chimed in, 'I just hope his aim is as good as he claims.' I was the one going under the drill so even though I had confidence in Dr Lee, I was now more nervous than I was before the meeting. This was going to be a tough twenty-four hours.

The key to successful DBS surgery is to place as many of the four DBS electrodes on each lead within the target structure as possible. This creates the largest stimulation pattern possible within the minuscule target area.

An accurate mapping of the brain and location of the STN and its orientation are paramount. The doctor uses Magnetic Resonance Imaging (MRI) to determine the three-dimensional coordinates of both STNs. Then the surgeon plots a path to the target area. The surgeon's journey through the brain is guided using micro-electroding, a technique that allows the surgeon to listen to the patient's brain *en route*. Apparently, a malfunctioning brain is noisy and loud in contrast to a normal functioning brain which does not have much to say. Finally, the specialists would periodically administer manual testing as additional security. Dr Lee was using every technique possible to ensure success.

In the pre-operation meeting, the representative from Abbot, Matthew Womack, demonstrated the equipment that would be implanted in the morning. One of the issues to be addressed was the power source for the transmitter, rechargeable or not. Matthew showed us an example of both. The trade-off was between size and longevity. The rechargeable was much bigger, but required few if any replacements. The recharging process was onerous and involved wearing a charging vest of sorts. What if I forgot or mislaid the charging connectors? The alternative was much sleeker and would protrude much less on my chest. I chose the smaller version. Matthew handed the nurse a sealed and sterile version of the neurotransmitter and lead package.

I would receive local anaesthetics at the site of the two holes and at the locations of the four bolts that would attach a metal halo to my skull. This was essentially a frame that would hold the drilling and insertion equipment. If the thought of screwing four bolts into your head like Frankenstein's Monster wasn't troublesome enough for you, the surgical team intended on bolting the head frame to the operating table. What a day we had in store!

After lunch, we went back to the clinic to have bloodwork done. We were also scheduled for a meeting with Dr Lee's surgical nurse. Ostensibly, the purpose was to get all the consent forms signed. I became a little perturbed when I was asked for a signed copy of my Durable Power of Attorney form, the one where Patty can turn off the machine if everything doesn't go well. I swallowed hard on that one.

At this stage I was tired and needed a rest, some time alone to process all I had heard.

I was distracted and anxious. A part of me wanted it to be over and strangely was ready to get the show going. I must encourage this internal voice. All that was required from me was to lie or sit there and allow Dr Lee to get on with it.

At dinner that night, I was quiet. My mind was churning. Then my phone rang. It was Harold, and true to his word, he had cleared his calendar and was here in Minnesota. His presence was reassuring and his familiarity with the procedure made us feel like insiders. He was the perfect tonic. That night, I fell asleep with no difficulty. The next morning, I woke to the usual neck struggles. Patty and I relied on our well-honed protocol: apply pressure to allow breathing and wear a moist warm neck heating pad. To alleviate the restlessness, I resorted to my morning shuffle. Only my right leg moved these mornings and then perhaps ten inches at a time without seemingly lifting off the ground. My left leg just pivoted, and as a result I made small circles in the room.

It was 5:15am and we had to be at St Mary's hospital at 6:00. My sister brought a wheelchair to the room, and I flopped into it after I was done shuffling. It was still dark when we got in our Uber for the one-mile ride. As we pulled under the hospital's covered front, I saw others who were in similar predicaments and wondered how many would undergo their procedures wide awake this morning. We waited in the appointed room, then Harold arrived. I refilled my reservoir of confidence which had dropped like shares in a stock market crash since after our arrival at the hospital.

Shortly after, Dr Lee came to say hello and met Harold. I thought perhaps he might ask Harold if he wanted to scrub in, but he didn't. This turned out to be a blessing as Harold kept three anxious women company for the next eight hours. Then the lead nurse took over. She had a big caring personality and could sense when I was getting weary or disconsolate. She held my hand at particularly tough moments and seemed to have a sixth sense for when an encouraging word or a smile was required.

It was 'go' time, and my trolley rolled down the corridor to the operating theatre. We passed a group of people whose backs were against the wall. They looked solemn, as if they were watching a funeral cortège go by. I recognised the Abbot representative, Matthew Womack. He and the others would be in the operating room too. He gave me a nod as we passed, but I was too slow or preoccupied to respond.

The operating room was impressive. It looked like this was its maiden voyage. It was spotless, super white and bright. The floors were shiny. First order of business, the nursing staff identified the exact spots where the four bolts would enter my skull and where local anaesthetic would be injected. I tried the frame on, and the staff marked the spots on my head. Then came the shots. I could feel the liquid numbing agent well up under the skin before finally dissolving. It must have absorbed quickly. Before I knew it, the industrial tools made an appearance, and the first bolt was being ratcheted into the bone on my left temple. It seemed to be taking an effort to make an impression in the bone as the nurse concentrated on his task, making little progress at first until finally gaining traction. It didn't hurt, but I felt it may at any moment. The next bolt was on the opposite side, catty-corner and out of my line of sight. Somehow, not being able to see made it easier to tolerate. I hoped this was a harbinger of how I would cope with the drilling process, all of which would happen outside my view finder.

Next up was to map the brain using an MRI in the theatre dedicated to this surgery. The halo sat on a platform on the MRI bed to ensure I kept steady. After less than twenty-five minutes my brain had been mapped, the STNs identified.

I was returned to the operating theatre, while Dr Lee and team calculated the precise X, Y and Z coordinates of the targets and the angle of entry to deliver an ideal lead orientation.

I was sitting up on a tilted bed as the nursing staff shaved my head in preparation for the two dime-sized holes that they were about to drill in my skull. With the extra weight of the frame, it was difficult to hold my head steady. I knew my head-nodding made their job more difficult. I felt like someone trying to stay awake at evening mass. Shortly, my movement would be restricted when they secured the frame to the table.

Being restrained in that manner took some resolution. Thank God, I didn't see all the contraptions that were attached to the head frame, nor did I feel the weight of the additional equipment. My head was firmly rooted to the table. The doctor used a high-speed drillbit to make the small hole in my skull. The drilling sounded worse than it felt. One tends to imagine pain when a drill gets close. I did feel the piercing of the dura matter, a thin layer of sensitive material under the skin. Think of the dura as a supertight swim cap. The dura is the one tissue in the brain that has pain sensors. The rest feels no pain when touched. So once through this outer protective layer, it is all motorway to the finish line.

Dr Lee used micro-electroding to listen to the brain. He had previously determined a target depth of 25mm. He instructed everyone in the operating theatre to be quiet, and we all listened as he gradually moved the stimulating electrode along the intended trajectory. We heard little except some background activity occasionally. He counted out loud in full numbers, 13 … 14. As he got closer to where he hoped the top of the STN was, he began counting in quarters 18.25 … 18.50 … 18.75. Still no activity then 19.25 … 19.50 … All of a sudden, it sounded like hundreds of unintelligible voices talking over each other like questions and answers with the prime minister in the British House of Parliament. We were in the correct zone, 23.0 still noisy … 23.25 a little quieter, and by 25 it was quiet again.

I survived the first wave, but I was a little unnerved. It's unimaginably scary to have people rummaging around in your brain. The lead nurse continued her kindness role. I frequently had a troubled look on my face, which she instantly recognised and bolstered my confidence with words of encouragement.

Next Dr Lee fed the Abbot lead through the same path as the micro electrode. Once in place the movement disorder specialists took over. The lead was attached to an external power source and current was introduced. At a power level of 1.1 mA, I experienced tingling in my legs and at 2.3 mA my speech began to slur. Based on these findings the lead was retracted by 0.5mm, and then the surgical team secured it in place.

It was then time for the other side. We had reached the target on the first try on the left. Would the team be as accurate the second time? If they were and I didn't get performance anxiety, we could be done over an hour ahead of schedule. That was enough motivation for me. It's a long time to convince yourself to stay relaxed. The drilling began again, and before I could even contemplate panic, Dr Lee was securing the right-side lead in place. He gathered up the excess wiring and left it under my scalp for later attachment to the transmitter. First time accurate placement on the right also. However, to be certain they took some scans. Dr Lee had more than lived up to expectations.

Enduring hardship often fosters a huge sense of achievement, particularly a hardship not many have encountered. The DBS survival club is not as exclusive as the sub-four-minute mile club, but the mental fortitude required is similar. I felt proud once we were through, and I wear my transmitter proudly like a winners' medal. I felt a huge sense of gratitude to Dr Lee and the entire surgical team. They treated me with the utmost kindness and respect and performed their duties expertly.

It was only in the recovery room that night that my thoughts turned to expectation for a great outcome. Until then, I had been in survival mode. Dr Lee kindly came by to check on me. The only complaint I had was the most debilitating headache I could imagine. And why not, given what I had been through. Dr Lee assured me this was normal. My sister Helen held an icebag on my head for most of the next twenty-four hours. I asked him how it was working with Abbot equipment. He seemed nonplussed about the technology change I had so timidly asked for, but did comment that the Abbot lead seemed very good at holding its course. I guess he meant the lead was stiffer. Either way it was buyer's confirmation for me. I spent one night in the hospital and was released the next day.

It was a long week as we waited for the second operation. I sat around looking for the honeymoon effect. I kept asking, 'Has anyone seen any improvement yet?'

It had snowed incessantly since we arrived, and someone had the idea that we should brave the snow to catch a musical recital at the local Catholic church. The church wasn't accessible via the underground labyrinth, so we ventured outside. I had a beanie over my gauze-encrusted and shaved head and was all bundled up in a wheelchair. There was so much snow it was difficult to tell where the pavement ended and the street began and it took all three of my companions to get me up over kerbs. We made the six blocks, but I can't say we enjoyed the recital much as we all had the return trip in the back of our minds.

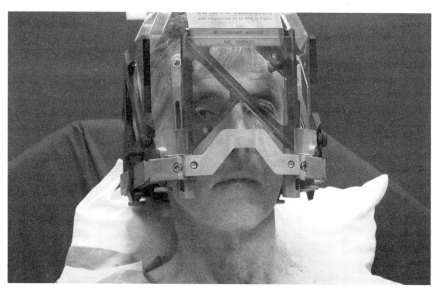

9 January 2019. Waiting nervously for the drilling to begin.

On day three after the surgery, I missed my third dose of Sinemet by over an hour and had no ill effects. It was the beginning of the longed-for honeymoon period. Three days later, in the neurotransmitter pre-operation meeting, Dr Lee seemed pleased with the effect I was experiencing. He instructed me to reduce my daily Sinemet intake by a third. The next day, Dr Lee successfully implanted the transmitter and tunnelled the wires under the skin and scalp to where he had temporarily stashed the excess wiring. He attached the two sets of wires, but we would have to wait another week to power up.

The honeymoon effect continued into week two as the snow continued to come down in buckets outside. My sisters left for Ireland early in the week. I was sorry to see them leave. It felt like the kids had gone back to school after summer break. Then my eldest son arrived, and all was right again in Minnesota.

The honeymoon effect lasted around ten days, and I had to return to my original dosage. All my symptoms came roaring back. I showed up for my initial programming session without my morning fill of Sinemet as directed. I must have demonstrated some lingering improvement as my UPDRS score was twenty-five and pre-surgery my score was fifty-one. My neurotransmitter was turned on. There were choices to be made: which of the four electrodes would be used, what amperage and frequency and which sector of each electrode. Initially at least, the specialists elected to treat the electrodes as if they were omni-directional. It made the process simpler.

There was improvement in both rigidity and tremors with current flowing on my left side. Unfortunately, my cramping became so intolerable that we had to discontinue right side programming and settle for default settings. After instruction on the handheld programmer, I was directed to raise the voltage incrementally to a pre-programmed level and told to return for a second programming session in six weeks.

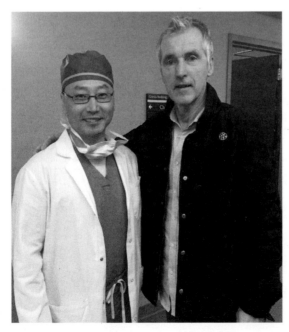

12 March 2019. Dr Kendall Lee, the surgeon with great precision.

## CHAPTER 16

# THERE ARE NO SHORTCUTS

There was an immediate return on investment in the form of a major reduction in neck cramping. Into the bargain I had reduced my Sinemet load to 1,000mg a day, which took the edge off the most obvious dyskinesia. Now it manifested as more of a rhythmic swaying. Unfortunately, progress screeched to a halt after the initial improvements. I compared my outcome with others I met. I spoke to one individual whose voltage was 6.2 mA. Maybe I needed higher settings.

I made two visits to the Mayo Clinic that spring for adjustments. The specialists said I looked better, and my body was much more still. The visit required another drug-free morning, which was again a challenge. There was the simple matter of my UPDRS score. Did my off-medicine score improve? This would be the litmus test for actual improvement. My score was twenty-four, a solid improvement from the fifty-one I had recorded before deep brain stimulation. Underneath the doubt, there was progress afoot. I tried to remain optimistic.

Programming an out-of-town patient can be challenging. A change can take a few days to fully bed in, making it difficult for the physician to completely achieve optimisation in the clinical setting. In two or three days, I would be back in Arkansas. The doctors had seemed to emphasise avoiding unintended consequences rather than achieving optimisation. Was that fear because I was remote? I understand they didn't want to send someone home, only to discover there are serious balance issues.

What about the home run? I had seen the videos of individuals turning off their transmitter and immediately experiencing severe tremors. The tremors disappeared as quickly once the device was turned back on. That immediacy was the benefit I expected.

The specialists had previously determined that electrode three on the right side and two on the left were ideal. These electrodes had the maximum therapeutic window and minimum side effects. On the second visit, they examined each of the three segments on both electrodes and determined that one of the three segments caused an undesirable side effect, namely the muscles on the left side of my mouth began to tighten. So, they turned off that segment and pushed the current to the other two segments only. They also increased the power to 2.3 mA on both sides.

They warned the new level was a significant increase and it would take my brain a while to adjust to it. After two weeks, I was instructed to raise the power settings in tiny increments of .05 to 2.7 mA on the left and 2.9 mA on the right. This should take about three more weeks. Allow a further two weeks for the changes to settle in and then return for further programming.

The doctors believed my walking problems were caused by 'peak dose dystonia'. The combination of stimulation and medicine was likely too much, and the resulting side effect, dystonia, was making me too stiff and rigid to walk. They advised I try a further reduction in Sinemet levels. The specialists advised patience and cautioned it would take time. I reminded myself to focus on the steps I controlled, turning up the voltage .05 mA at a time for example. That was how I could influence the outcome.

The surgery had gone as well as we expected. I experienced a definite honeymoon effect, and there was substantial relief from the incessant neck cramps. Why did the momentum stop? I suspected that closer supervision was required. We needed real-time feedback and adjustment.

It also had become clear to clinic staff that a more hands-on approach was essential to maximise the benefit of my surgery. We agreed to transfer responsibility for optimisation to Dr Dhall at UAMS. Dr Dhall was more accessible and the more changes you make the more monitoring you need. This was clearly going to take some time.

Often you apply a big push when a nudge may have sufficed. Think of Shackleton, Crean, McCarthy and the other three men who left Elephant Island hoping to navigate to South Georgia Island, eight hundred miles away in an endless ocean. If they missed, it meant their demise and that of twenty-two others depending on them. The slightest early course adjustment would keep them on target. Conversely, a tiny mistake in calculation would compound over eight hundred miles and could be the difference between rescue or perishing.

There are major benefits in getting the basics right in any endeavour. This is especially so in the small-business arena. My father was a serial entrepreneur and owned numerous businesses during his lifetime. On my long-form birth certificate his occupation is listed as potato merchant. Apparently, he bought potatoes in bulk and prepared and sold them to restaurants and hotels. Before that, he owned and operated threshing machines for hire to local farmers. In between these two businesses, he owned and managed a pub in Limerick City. By my third birthday, he was no longer in the potato business, he had started what became a successful soft-drinks bottling business called Shannon Minerals.

In those days there were no large grocery stores, instead towns were dotted with little shops. People bought meat at the butcher's, greens from the fruit and vegetable bloke and bread from a baker. My father's business served these small shops with two trucks. Cash was the most common payment method. The coins that the drivers collected accumulated back at the office for a few weeks or more until the bag took two hands to lift. Oddly, my father would then bring it home for the family to count.

I clearly remember my brother and eventually my twin sisters joining in. On occasions our good friends, the Brownes, were included in the counting. My mother would summon us to the kitchen where a couple of heavy, cloth bags lay on the table. My dad would empty the contents onto the kitchen table. The massive pile contained all denominations of silver coins and a lot of halfpenny and penny coins. Everyone vied for the silver coin shift, the half shilling, or 6p, and the shilling. This was before Ireland changed its currency to the decimal system.

The instructions provided by my father were easy to follow. All the coins were counted in stacks of ten. Each counter was assigned a coin, rummaged around until they had a pile of their assigned coin and created stacks of ten. Counting was monotonous, and sometimes we resorted to stacking. Establish one stack of ten and eyeball subsequent stacks against it. You could lop off any excess or add to if you were short. My father discouraged this practice as pure laziness and insisted that every stack be a counted one.

My father enjoyed the perks of seniority and was the bagger. He would grab five stacks and put them in small paper bags provided by the bank. These bags were put in the cloth bags for transport to the Bank of Ireland. We were all eager to participate in the counting routine and raced each other counting stacks.

I went to the bank with my father to lodge the money once. I had wondered how the bank verified that the correct amount was actually in each bag. They used a fairly prehistoric looking weighing scale, at least by today's terms. The bank teller put the appropriate number of bags on the scale and checked in his official bank notebook what five pounds in pennies should weigh in pounds and ounces.

The scale used was analogue, and as the platform with the weight of the appropriate number of coins depressed, an arrow moved clockwise around the dial and settled uneasily on a number. I remember that indicator quivering for a good four or five seconds after it had chosen its final resting spot. The teller squatted down to peer at the still vibrating appendage to determine the correct reading. He then cross-checked that reading against the number in the standards book and declared the number of coins on the scale accurate or inaccurate. Any suspected deficiency was addressed instantly, bags were opened, and a manual count performed. This happened rarely according to my dad.

The next time we were gathered for the count, I used the stacking technique openly. I counted an accurate stack of ten to use as the template and began assembling bundles into what felt like ten. Then I crouched down to deploy the eyeball exam as I scanned from the template to the uncounted stacks.

I was caught in a flash, 'Francis, what the devil are you doing?'

'I am making stacks of ten, Dad.'

'I instructed you to count stacks of ten, didn't I?'

'But the bank fellow only weighed the bags on that old scale. How would he tell if I got the odd one wrong?'

'That's not the point. I certify the amount is accurate, so it needs to be.'

'Oh, come on, Dad.'

'Absolutely not. I said count, and we will count.'

That was the end of guesstimating.

I suspect if my father had lived longer, he may have explained what, if anything, he hoped to achieve from this bi-monthly exercise. It may have simply been free labour, but surely there was an underlying message. Naturally, he wanted to teach us the value of money, after all it was mostly small coins and wouldn't total more than a few hundred pounds at a time. I imagine he was telling us to look after the pennies, and the pounds will look after themselves.

In my first programming visit with Dr Dhall, we spent the best part of three hours together. First, he saved the current settings so that if anything we tried backfired, we could revert to them for relief. He made two major changes. On the right body side, he changed the pulse width from 60 to 80 MHz. On the left side, he eliminated a segment on a lower level and added a segment on a second level. This com pletely changed the area of stimulation.

Over the next year, we made multiple adjustments as Dr Dhall tried new frequencies, new segments and more stimulation. I saw steady but slow improvement. I continued to track each hour of the day and provide detailed feedback on each modification. Dr Dhall had increased the stimulation levels to 3.45 on the left side and 3.55 on the right. Still, we hadn't reached optimisation. Dr Dhall cautioned that more amperage isn't always the solution.

Then Dr Dhall introduced a new drug called Gocovri, which promised to be a catalyst for acceleration of benefits. Gocovri is an extended-release version of the agonist Amantadine. This drug turned out to be central to any sustained improvement. The unexpected benefits provoked by Gocovri caused Dr Dhall to consider lowering the levels.

He called on a colleague at UAMS for assistance. Dr Virmani manages the gait analysis lab. This lab has a fifteen-metre walking mat with numerous cameras at ankle height. The patient wears multiple sensors on different body parts. The first pass is performed with the stimulation turned off. Then stimulation is turned up in 0.5 mA increments until your gait begins to deteriorate. The computer then works its magic, and the ideal level of stimulation is derived for the first side. The neurologist in charge of your care then decides the appropriate levels given the other symptoms.

I was scheduled for a follow-up session to hone the results, but then Covid-19 wrecked that plan. People all over the world were instructed to stay at home, wear masks, and limit guests to their homes. Offices shut down, weddings were cancelled, funerals were unattended, and the elderly left unvisited. And, worst of all, millions lost their lives. Elective medical procedures were cancelled as was my gait analysis. Many of us didn't leave our homes for months on end. I had grown accustomed to being housebound.

Dr Virmani used his experience to interpret the outcome of the incomplete study. He estimated that my optimum level on the left side should be lowered to 2.7 mA. Fortunately, the reduction was within the prescribed and pre-programmed range on my iPod remote device. I made the adjustments from home over a video call. Now both sides were at 2.7 mA. Gradually the improvements compounded, and my reliance on Sinemet dramatically decreased. I now take 400mg a day and have little, if any, dyskinesia.

It took two years to experience the entire improvement that deep brain stimulation had to offer. I had been forewarned that it may take that long, but I was too preoccupied with surviving the surgery to digest. I heard 'wide awake for five hours' and tuned everything else out. The improvement had been generated by numerous factors working in symphony, the settings on my transmitter, the medicine and a specific exercise programme designed to address my weaknesses.

I left nothing to chance in creating a strength and conditioning programme. I called on my friend and therapist, Ger Hartmann, who flew from Ireland, accompanied by another friend, Ian Bolger, to assess and design a programme.

Over a week, he identified my gait issues and exercises to address the underlying cause. The problem was weak glute and hip muscles. Mine was caused by a lack of signalling which caused a paucity of activity resulting in weakness. If we strengthened that area, then we could compensate for the wiring shortcomings. At the very least we would slow the regression. I can't say that my walking has improved greatly, but it is serviceable.

The problem with exercise is our old friend, expectations. We are accustomed to exercise generating positive results. We exercise to improve our health. This is not the case with exercise and Parkinson's. You work out with no hope for improvement. The best you can hope for is to stem the tide, slow the steady advancement of the disease. I have trouble reconciling this reality. There is no reward, no payoff. You don't know the disease timeline so how can you be sure that all that sweating and showering made a difference? Then there is the question, is there some increased payoff for working even harder?

You have to trust that there is some benefit. I have never heard of a circumstance where inactivity was productive except in recovery from an injury. I am hard-wired to trust in the healing elements of exercise. I find that when I am having a bad day, thirty minutes on the treadmill gives me a boost and at least distracts me from my condition.

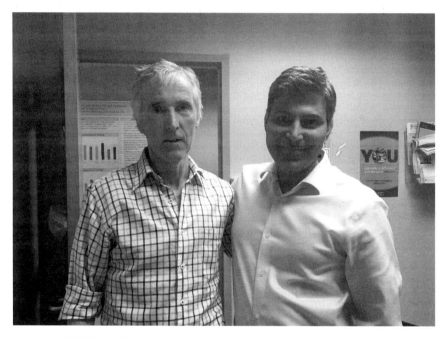

2 August 2019. Dr Rohit Dhall, the movement disorder specialist who rescued me.

## CHAPTER 17

# BE PREPARED TO GO IT ALONE

Parkinson's throws a depth charge into your life and one consequence is your reliance on others to do what were once inconsequential tasks. Such reliance can be humbling, but when you finally shake off the stubbornness and accept help, you reclaim some of your former life. It really does take a team to deal with the realities of Parkinson's.

My team is primarily made up of Patty and my three sons. One is usually nearby watching and waiting to assist. There are some good friends who I can rely on to take me to lunch; attentive enough that Patty will trust them. But not everyone is suited to caregiving. It's not for a lack of caring; they simply don't know how to interact with you.

I have had many teammates in the past in both work and athletics, but it is a college relay team that highlights the need for all to be singing from the same hymnal. It was 1981, and I was a civil engineering student at the University of Arkansas. At the age of seventeen, when I left secondary school, I had no idea what line of work I would ultimately pursue. I just knew I wanted to run in circles until I figured the future out.

I had intended to enrol in architecture, but that programme required lab classes that lasted until 5pm. Track practice began at 3:30pm. This presented a clear problem; the track coach would not make an exception or change practice. So, I changed to civil engineering, the closest discipline to architecture. Nonetheless, in the engineering programme there were a couple of classes that overlapped with track practice. Namely, a surveying class that was only offered in the spring of a student's third year. Unless I could finish early or my training group agreed to wait for me, I was on my own for workouts that semester.

That spring, Arkansas was set to compete at Franklin Field in Philadelphia in the Penn Relays. Over the prior four or five years, Arkansas had been dominant at southern and midwest relay meetings, namely the Kansas and Texas Relays and the Drake Relays which arguably rivals Penn. We would be matched against Villanova in their hometown. The best Irish athletes had previously attended Villanova, and now there were a number of us at this southern upstart school. Villanova had some of the finest milers in NCAA history such as Eamonn Coghlan, Ronnie Delany and Marty Liquori and had a legendary coach named Jumbo Elliott.

Their current star and anchor of their relays was a South African, Sydney Maree. He was older than most of his peers. He was twenty-six, and a world-class athlete who would have been in contention for world titles had it not been for apartheid, which prohibited South Africans from international competition until the 1992 Olympics in Barcelona. Additionally, Villanova was riding a seventeen-year victory streak in the distance medley relay and a similarly impressive run in the 4 x 1,500m relay.

Practice had extra significance that week. Everyone was excited about our first trip to Penn. Each of my three teammates was confident they could match the credentials of anyone on their legs. Anyone who is familiar with relay running understands that it generally comes down to the anchor – or final – leg. There was no denying that it would result in a Maree versus

O'Mara match-up. The week rushed by and the trepidation multiplied, not due to the intimidation factor, but due to the heightened expectations of our team. I could sense everyone was thinking, 'I don't know about the rest of you, but I got my man.' Not being at practice, I could not modulate expectations. There was no voice of reason, just runaway optimism. Good workouts fuelled the fire, and by the time I finished my surveying assignment and arrived at practice, they were essentially practising press interviews. It was just a matter of showing up, and we would be awarded the Championship of America trophy.

All the pressure was on me. True, my teammates could hold their own with the opponents on the earlier legs and could perhaps run a slightly faster leg, but there was no way I would have a sufficiently large gap to hold off Maree. I couldn't live up to their expectations. My personal best for the 1,500m was 3:40.36, Maree's best was 3:35.00.

Throughout the remainder of the week, I watched as my teammates' confidence grew. We travelled to Philly on Thursday, which meant missing two days of college that week and required me to bring my schoolbooks. This further exacerbated the tension. It was impossible to study and impossible to prepare for Villanova.

The next day, Friday, was the first of three relays I ran that weekend. There was rain in the forecast and a slight chill in the air as we drove past the University of Pennsylvania campus and approached the venerable old stadium. The atmosphere was chaotic. There was a massive heaving crowd attempting to get beyond the street vendors. There were the yellow and green colours of the Jamaican flag, and the smell of Caribbean food in the air. There was nowhere to park and nowhere to warm up. What a mess! I saw some Villanova tracksuits. Apparently, they had taken a thirty-minute train ride from mainline in the suburbs of Philadelphia, so they weren't urgently looking for a parking spot.

We convinced the coach to drop us off, while he found a spot. For some reason Sam Frees, the university's swim coach, had travelled separately to the meet and had figured out the entry protocol, so we followed him. Inside was even crazier than outside. Penn offers multiple categories of each event; there are over 100 heats of the 4 x 400m alone. So, to say they are punctilious would be grossly understating their efficiency.

The hectic environment dampened some of my teammates' confidence, but they were still talking a great game. We warmed up, jogging cautiously amongst the crowd, dodging errant kids and people darting out of bathrooms. We stretched and did some sprints. All of a sudden, we were on.

Coach was frantic. 'Come on, come on, they are calling the Distance Medley.'

We weren't moving at a satisfactory pace for Coach. This time we could sense the urgency in his voice. 'They will seriously start without you. Come on. Just carry your racing shoes. You can put them on in the pen.'

He had to give last-minute instructions to us as a group as we dashed through the crowds to the check-in area. 'We're going to win this, lads.'

He turned to me and said, 'If they give you a lead, you need to bring it home. Don't mess it up.'

I'm sure in different circumstances, he would have given me better instructions. There was simply not enough time. We were all rookies that day. To say I was overwhelmed would be generous. The occasion got to me. There were multiple pens for staging. There was one to check your number and another to check the order you intended to race. You advanced through the pens as your race got closer. The pens were underneath the crowded stands. It was loud and intimidating. I could hear the crowd swell with excitement and groan with disappointment, while feet pounded on the bleachers above us.

We were moved to the first of two track-side pens and separated by running order, all the lead-off runners together. I was standing within feet of the great Sydney Maree. The drizzle turned to rain as we were herded into the next pen. These pens are roped-off enclosures that force you to walk back and forth much like a present-day TSA line at an airport. Inevitably, you encounter the same individual multiple times as you weave toward the start. The huge crowd was buzzing. The red brick wall that surrounds the oval glistened on the wet track. I tried to take it all in, but I kept running into the seemingly unflappable Maree. How often can you feign confidence let alone indifference?

The lead-off athletes were on the starting line, and they were off. We were in the mix. The rain came down a little harder. Our second leg kept us in it and handed off in contention. After the hand-off to the third leg, the anchors were released from the pen and free to loosen their legs after spending the last thirty minutes in a stockyard. Our third leg was doing exceptionally well, and it appeared to be the Razorbacks versus the Wildcats. I was even going to have a lead.

I took the baton from my teammate. I had about a thirty-metre lead, but I was being chased by one of the world's best. I heard the roar of the home crowd when he took the hand-off. It was deafening as he set off in pursuit of me. As you can imagine by now, he mowed me down as did two or three others. I don't believe I would have beaten him on a good day that year, but the truth is, I grossly underperformed.

My teammates were shocked. They had worked themselves into a frenzy, and there was one person to blame. I had botched it, but even if I hadn't, was it reasonable to heap all these expectations on one man? My coach was no different. He too allowed his disappointment to boil over into anger. At my most vulnerable, standing trackside in the rain, soaked to the skin, they all gave me the cold shoulder. They got in the cars to return to the hotel and left me alone at the track. It was petty of them. Nonetheless, there I was wallowing in self-pity.

The swim coach who was spectating saw me beaten down and abandoned and gave me a ride to the hotel. While I showered, he washed and dried my racing gear. He took me to dinner that night and gave me a pep talk. He was a big demonstrative man and was one hell of a motivator. He described how to turn defeat and disappointment into determination and if you're lucky, rage. Bottle it up and use it as fuel. I can't say for certain whether the team and coach excluded me from dinner, or I chose to avoid them. Not that I was embarrassed, I was over that. I was now angry.

The next day was bright and clear, as was my head. I was focused on giving it my all, not on revenge over Maree or vindication to my teammates or coach, but for me. Giving less than your best can be soul sucking. I had tasted that plenty the previous day. I now had to right the ship before it grounded. Whatever happened today, Sydney Maree was going to know he was in a battle.

I ran into my coach as I was leaving breakfast.

'You got home from the track alright yesterday, then?' he asked.

'It was fine. I managed to get a lift.'

'I told Sam to hang around and take care of you,' Coach said.

'Oh, thanks,' I replied.

'You're anchoring again today.'

Strangely I hadn't given a change in the line-up a thought, but I guess it was understandable that he'd consider it.

'Sorry about yesterday, Coach,' was all I could manage.

He merely said, 'You're better than yesterday, kid.'

He always called you 'kid' when you were in favour. Sam Frees must have reported back how devastated I had been and how determined I was to make amends.

'I'll give him everything I got today. I'll make him work for it.'

'I know you will, kid.'

That was the totality of the instructions I got or, for that matter, needed. That day's relay was the 4 x 1,500 metre, and the two primary contenders were Villanova and Arkansas. Everyone predicted we would gap the field, and then it would be a shootout between anchors. There was quite a shock in the stadium when the line-ups were announced. I reckon everyone assumed I would be demoted to one of the earlier legs or replaced entirely. Doubtless, my confidence had been shattered by Maree, and I would capitulate too easily.

True to form after the first two legs, Villanova and Arkansas had put some distance on the rest of the field. When the third leg had a lap remaining, I shouted at our runner who was in second place sitting on their runner. 'Stay right there, you're perfect!'

There's two hundred to go, and we are still in perfect position. It is paramount in a relay to not give your anchor a sucker lead, especially in a two-man contest. The runner behind has a huge advantage.

Better to make Maree take the lead, do all the work and mount an attack on the last lap. This was turning out perfectly. Maree would get the baton two metres ahead and would have to run blind the whole way. But then it went awry. Our third man decided to show Franklin Field patrons that he had the better kick. He launched himself into a mad sprint and gave me an eight-metre lead over Maree, a completely pointless gesture that established nothing.

What could I do to shake him off? Nothing really. I knew he was faster than me. I decided to run a moderate pace and rebuff any move for the front. I had the lead, and I was determined to make him earn it. I set off at a semi-honest pace, and he caught me before the back straight. Then he simply sat on me, happy in the knowledge that he had comfortably dealt with me the prior day. Everyone in the stadium was waiting for his big move, anticipating, almost relishing the moment. The stadium with some 45,000 people in attendance was eerily silent. All I could hear was the sound of his untroubled breathing and his shoes hitting the track. Over the silence, I could hear my coach screaming.

Coming to the bell, the crowd's response alerted me that Sydney had begun his patented push for home. He tried to surge into the lead as we approached the finish line. My plan was to deny him the lead for as long as I could. We were both sprinting as we crossed the line with a lap to go. I rebuffed him and kept the crazed pace going as Maree gathered himself for his next push. The crowd was wild with excitement as we charged down the back straight. At the halfway mark on that last lap, 200m left, he launched another bid for the front; but I matched his effort again and held him off. This time he kept sprinting, but he was on the outside with further to run. Around the last turn we ran side by side, both of us straining for the lead. The crowd was roaring now, fully engrossed in the contest. We drove into the final straight, still neck and neck, and continued our tussle through the finishing line. I closed my eyes as we both pushed those final metres and opened them to a 'Well done, man' from Maree. He had won by the narrowest of margins … one hundredth of a second. The last lap took a little over fifty seconds.

My teammates surrounded me on the infield as the crowd applauded. It was a strange circumstance. You realise, that even surrounded by friends and teammates, your only company is your shadow. The decision to knuckle down and confront a dilemma is yours and yours alone. Only you can decide if your response is flight or fight.

It's no different with Parkinson's. Although you are surrounded by family, you have to bear the cross yourself. Nobody can take your place. Struggling through an off period can be a challenge. All you can do is grin and bear it. Company is generally comforting, but sometimes you have to shut out the world.

While a loved one or friend cannot bear the burden, they can relieve pressure by taking care of daily necessities: paying bills, ensuring tuition has been looked after and Christmas presents bought. In moments of Parkinson's-induced anxiety, having something to actually worry about would be insufferable.

I have surmised that much of the benefit ultimately comes from a reduction in Sinemet. I had decreased my dosage from sixteen to eight pills a day after six months. I was determined to gradually wean myself to a lower dose. A year and a half later I was back to 100mg tablets and had further reduced my dosage to one pill every four hours or 400mg a day. Easy to remember: 8am, noon, 4pm and 8pm. I have flirted with three tablets a day and it almost worked. I intend another assault on three soon. It's my way of letting Parkinson's know that I am not going to fold.

Another apparent victory for Parkinson's was my inability to visit my homeland. Being Irish is very important to me and getting home is essential. All my family live there and life-long friends too. Four years into my Parkinson's journey, my condition discouraged me from making the all-day trip home. I was fortunate to have many friends and family members who

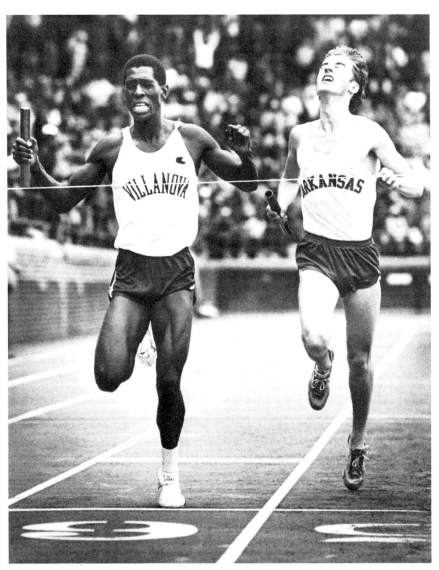

25 April 1981. A crushing defeat by Sydney Maree at the Penn Relays.

were prepared to come my way. Two and a half years after deep brain stimulation, I was well enough to make my first trip to Ireland in eight years. The main concern was my reactions to jetlag. Sleep is vital to cope with Parkinson's, and a bad night's sleep generally results in a miserable day. My secondary concern was how I would fare in two challenges Ger Hartmann had planned for me. These challenges had motivated me to work on my strength and conditioning throughout the spring.

I did manage to sleep around five hours on the flight and arrived excited to be home and looking forward to both challenges. I completed a ten-kilometre paddle on a two-man kayak with Ger doing the majority of the work. The highlight of the trip was a wonderful country house we rented in Kerry where my mother is from. It was a one-hundred and fifty-year-old house on Kenmare Bay where we hosted my siblings for three nights and some old teammates from the University of Arkansas the rest of the week. I even managed to make a quick visit to the South Pole, the pub once owned by that hero of mine, the Antarctic explorer, Tom Crean.

## CHAPTER 18

# ONE STEP AT A TIME

I have been fascinated with polar exploration ever since my childhood visit to Tom Crean's pub. Men of that era were tougher and more determined than the majority of us. Even with all our comforts today, a trip to the polar region is still not a cakewalk. I always wanted to see for myself how grim and foreboding the Antarctic can be. Perhaps my intent was to reprise any inspiration gained there in battles yet to come.

My health had improved further since my excursions in Ireland during the summer, and I decided it was now or never. I asked my friend Marcus O'Sullivan to accompany me, and he accepted the challenge. Marcus, like me, is a Tom Crean devotee and is a distant relative of Tim McCarthy, the Cork man who was also a member of Shackleton's crew on his ship, *Endurance*. Marcus has made *Endurance* required reading for the captains of his track teams at Villanova University.

Marcus was reluctant at first. Accommodating his coaching schedule was paramount, so we had to find an expedition with availability during the holidays. His other concern was how much care I would need. Not that he was unwilling; he wanted to be certain he could manage. The last time he had seen me was eighteen months prior, and at that juncture, I had yet to experience the complete healing power of the surgery. I assured him I was substantially better. I was getting around fine. I actually had followed up my hiking endeavours in Ireland with numerous three-mile walks. Nonetheless, he wanted to speak with Patty, who told him I was good to go, but that I may have some freezing issues at night and may require an arm while hiking.

Patty told him that I tend to overestimate what I can do and that he may need to be the voice of reason on occasion. She also told him that I had been talking about the Antarctic too long, and if it were not for crossing the Drake Passage twice, she would go too. The mention of the passage grabbed his attention. He wanted to know more about this impediment. The Drake Passage is a five-hundred-mile stretch between the tip of South America, Cape Horn, and the Antarctic. It is purportedly the most turbulent water in the world. Naturally, he searched for the Drake Passage on the web and not surprisingly was directed to YouTube videos of giant waves engulfing the bows of ships as they rode the enormous swells. That was enough to scare anyone. On top of spending four days and a thousand nautical miles feeling like you were churning around in a washing machine, you had to spend a day flying to Ushuaia, Argentina, the southernmost city in the world. It was an ordeal, to be fair.

My mobile rang the following day, and it was Marcus. 'Hey, did you know about this Drake Passage?'

I knew this was more than a simple inquiry. There was a wave of trepidation behind that question. So, no point in an elaborate answer.

'I did,' I said.

I knew I just had to listen.

'I just got through watching videos. Have you watched any?' Before I could respond he asked, 'Have you seen the size of the waves?'

I reminded him that there were patches for seasickness and that the videos online were most likely taken in winter, and we would be there in summer. I could tell I hadn't convinced him when he related a story about crossing the Irish Sea on a car ferry as a teenager. The boat encountered choppy waters and most on board got ill.

'… and that was the Irish Sea … in the summer,' he recounted.

I offered encouragement. 'Here's how I see it. All explorers went through the Drake. It's the price of entry. If it was easy to get there every Tom, Dick and Harry would be on their way.'

'Not always true. You can cross from Western Australia.'

'But Shackleton, McCarthy and Crean went from South America.'

'Fair enough.' The penny had dropped. It was time to reinforce.

'We will be on the same waters as the *Endurance*. It'll be worth it.'

Marcus was rightly concerned about the level of care I would require. We talk frequently, and he has become my most loyal and dependable friend. The last time we met was at an indoor track meet in Boston. I was doing much better at the time, but I hardly appeared ready to make an arduous trip to the Antarctic. I needed help getting around and was constantly leaning on others for safety.

We were planning an expedition on a twelve-day National Geographic voyage that was due to leave Ushuaia, Argentina for the Antarctic Peninsula on 28 December. We expected to spend four days traversing the Drake Passage and the remainder exploring the Antarctic with hiking, and zodiac and kayaking excursions twice daily. Add to that a strenuous mixture of freezing temperatures and ice and snow and his anxiety was merited.

The brochure describing the expedition gave it a strenuous rating for activity. Marcus was more worried when we were asked for a doctor to vouch for our fitness to participate on a very official looking form. I wasn't certain my general practice doctor would approve. I drove to his office and very sheepishly asked the nurse if she would have the doctor attest that I was fit for Antarctic duty.

Another mandate was received from the voyage operator. Each guest was required to obtain emergency evacuation insurance. The Antarctic is a remote and unwelcoming environment, and if an injury occurs, there is almost nothing that can be done for the injured. The ship has a doctor on board, but a serious injury would necessitate airlifting at considerable expense.

The doctor's office called me. Everything seemed to conspire against us getting to the polar region. I was certain the doctor was calling to tell me this was not my greatest idea and declining to attest to my preparedness. Instead, it was the nurse calling to say the forms were ready for pick-up. I picked up those forms that same afternoon for fear he may have a change of heart. He had written a note saying he had no doubt that I could manage anything I encountered and to enjoy.

My doctor was convinced I could cope. Now I just had to convince Marcus.

Eventually, Marcus spoke to our therapist friend, Ger Hartmann, who delineated the adventures he had led me on that summer. The ten-kilometre kayaking trip on Lough Derg and the two serious hikes, the latter being the climb up Moylussa. I must admit that I was joined on both hikes by former track friends who did everything short of carry me up the steep sections. Nonetheless, I did manage to summit. Marcus would have to shoulder the responsibility, but Ger eased his concerns with a reminder to take regular rests.

With Marcus finally on board, we began planning the gear required for a polar visit. Temperatures were expected to be between -25C and -10C. Layered clothing was recommended to deal with the cold. The body is like a constant mini furnace with 39C output, so all you need is to retain that heat. Layering clothing provides multiple pockets of warm air that insulate the body. We had plenty of relevant experience with layering and shedding of gear from our running days. Marcus, who is still very heavily involved in track and who lives in the cold northeast, took responsibility for acquiring the appropriate equipment.

There was also the issue of seasickness. That was a responsibility that we were both determined to address. We ended up with all manner of motion medication from the industrial solution patches to the slightly more common Dramamine to the homeopathic, ginger drops to ginger chewing gum. We had a full arsenal.

We were finally all in. We just had to avoid contracting Covid-19 before departure. This was no easy task with the Omicron variant raging across the world and the huge swathe of the population not vaccinated. We had to be super vigilant around the holidays. Marcus even cancelled a recruiting trip to Ireland to preclude the potential for infection.

We arranged to meet in Atlanta and catch the same connecting flight to Miami. The plan was for Patty to get me on the flight to Atlanta, and Marcus to meet me at the gate after his flight from Philly and help me to our next flight. He was surprised to see how much I had improved in eighteen months. I was walking with relative ease. I had devised a surrogate walking aid, a rolling backpack on four wheels. With the handle fully extended, it acted like a hyper steady cane and combated the uncertainty in my gait.

We made our way to the next gate with ease. Challenges seem to bring out the best in me and the prospect of this epic journey had inspired me to work hard on my strength and conditioning in the previous few months. I needed that preparation for the journey ahead.

After a night in Miami, and a successful pre-boarding rapid antigen Covid test, we were on board a charter flight for the southernmost city in the world, Ushuaia, Argentina. The overnight flight landed at noon the next day after flying over the rough but imperious looking peaks of Tierra del Fuego. We emerged into the bright sunshine that is rare in that part of the world. Ushuaia is more typically resplendent in its dreariness than in warm sun, but the guide warned that can change in an inkling.

As if on cue, it began to drizzle just enough to create chatter among fellow passengers, all of whom were distracted by the impending crossing of the Drake Passage. We entered the harbour and boarded the *National Geographic Explorer*, a small but sturdy looking exploration ship that held sixty guests, sixty crew and eight naturalists with *National Geographic*. We were welcomed by the captain and the exploration leader. Everyone seemed to have noticed the increased wind on the bay, and the conversation invariably centred on when was the appropriate time to indulge in a seasickness patch. A passenger advised that the patch can compromise your balance and not to take it until you absolutely must. Another countered that taking it then is too late because of the absorption time. And then out of the blue, somebody alerted us that the body of water we were presently on was not in fact the Drake Passage but the Beagle Channel. We were apparently hours from the Passage. Whoa … what was it like out there in open water?

We began to explore the ship. It has a special bow to break ice and stabilisers to quell the rolling motion of the water. It was evident that the ship was prepared for poor conditions. The dining room furniture was fastened to the floors. The chairs in the lounge were permanently secured to the floor on a single pedestal and the phrase 'one hand for the ship and one hand for yourself' was emblazoned on placards on most walls.

The Drake Passage is the body of water between Cape Horn in Chile at the tip of South America and the South Shetland islands that sit on top of the Antarctic Peninsula. It is the convergence point of the Atlantic, Pacific and Southern Oceans, and since the currents here have no nearby landmass to interfere, they are the choppiest waters in the world. They make getting to the Antarctic difficult, but anything worth achieving is generally out of arm's reach. If the journey isn't worth the trouble, the destination may not be worth the effort.

We pulled anchor and motored down the Beagle Channel. The entire group assembled for the standard 'abandon ship' drills. The expedition leader noted the distracted countenance on each of our faces and instantly recognised the perpetrator, the Drake Passage. He delivered the best new year's gift possible. For the outbound trip at least, swells would be a highly manageable two to three metres. It would be what old hands referred to as the Drake Lake. Some passengers regretted having patches already on, but all were grateful for the good news.

After the long flight to Ushuaia, we settled in for a solid night's sleep. We entered the Drake Passage a little before midnight and the swaying began. Fortunately, our cabin was in the middle of the ship, and we experienced less of a roller-coaster ride and more of a soothing effect. (That's what we convinced ourselves of at least.) Those whose cabins were further out on the pendulum had a much different experience. Two-to-three-metre swells are not trivial after all.

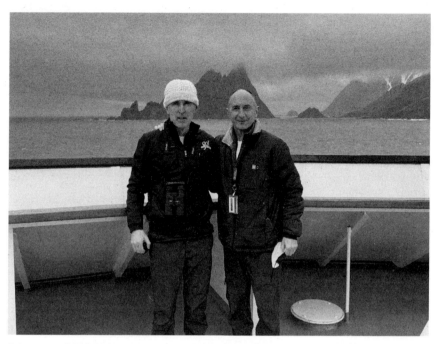

I January 2022. With Marcus as Elephant Island looms in the background.

We woke to wonderful news; we had made great progress in the relatively benign conditions and were making tracks toward an unexpected treat, Elephant Island, famous in *Endurance* lore. This forlorn lump of lava is the spot where Shackleton, after being trapped on the ice on the Antarctic for two winters, left twenty-two of his men under two overturned lifeboats as he and five others headed off on an eight-hundred-mile journey to South Georgia Island in search of rescue. Frank Wild was left in charge and managed to buoy the remaining crew members' mood for four months until Shackleton's return to rescue them. Tom Crean and Tim McCarthy accompanied Shackleton on that monumental journey, navigating by night with no instruments across the Drake. Tomorrow morning, coincidentally four days before the hundredth anniversary of Shackleton's death, we would be at Camp Wild on Elephant Island.

With great anticipation we managed to whittle away another day on the high seas with some card playing, and when the seas cooperated, lectures from the naturalists in the lounge. My balance, already compromised, was especially challenged in these tempestuous waters. The ropes and railings were a great assistance, but frankly I had so little control over the outcome of each step, I stayed put in the cabin and watched the lectures on closed-circuit television. There was one benefit of the rolling motion. I could use the forward rolling of the ship to propel me upward from a seated or prostrate position. Every cloud has a silver lining, I guess.

We woke in the morning to a communication from the expedition leader that we would be at Elephant Island shortly after breakfast. The waters were calmer here on the lee side of the Island. We made our way along this lonely scrap of rock jutting out of the darkest blue ocean. It was treeless and weathered. It was no place for man or beast, except for those men who had no other option when marooned there for a desperate four months in 1916.

They had previously spent two awful winters squashed in the polar ice. They salvaged three rescue boats, shoring them up with wood from the *Endurance,* and dragged them across the ice floe, subsequently rowing and sailing, when winds cooperated, in search of habitation. They ended up on this uninhabitable mound of volcanic rock. Amazingly, they endured in that environment for four full months. Nobody was lost or left behind; every single crew member survived.

Our captain stalled the motor just off the shore. Marcus and I were on the deck as we approached. We scanned the shoreline until we saw the monument honouring Frank Wild. We stared in wonder at the daunting sight. We took pictures with the craggy coast in the background as the ship dallied there for over an hour. As predicted, the water was far too choppy to attempt landings in zodiacs, so we had to be content with staring through binoculars. Not much had changed about this unfriendly place since those anguished men had braved the crashing waves a century before.

We cruised around the island for over two hours, confirming that there was no vegetation, water, nor shelter anywhere. We saw Cape Valentine where the men first came ashore. This spot was even more forsaken than the place they ultimately chose. After about two hours on deck in the numbing cold, we had imbibed all the destituteness we could consume and went inside to warm ourselves.

The ship motored on to our ultimate destination, the Antarctic, where I would test myself. I had prepared well and was eager for the challenge. *National Geographic* expeditions typically involve two off-boat excursions a day. First you disembark the ship on to zodiacs and then either go ashore or remain on the zodiac for tours on the water. Two landings contained epic hikes. The first was to a cairn on the highest point on the western end of Booth Island. The second was a hike to the ridge at Orne Harbor. Adding degrees of complexity to both of these hikes was the elevation gain, two feet of crunchy snow, inappropriate footwear and subzero temperatures.

I was experiencing freezing episodes again, but I was determined to reach the summit of both hikes. I imagine the travel and balance challenge of the swaying ship contributed to symptoms. The freezing was especially evident in the evening. On a number of occasions, Marcus had to help me get ready for bed, and in one instance, had to get me into bed.

I had expected that we would chat till all hours of the night like we did in our athletic days when we roomed together. Back then we could have talked for Ireland, let alone run for the island. We did develop some interesting sleep habits, idiosyncrasies you might say, that I noticed Marcus had not divested. He uses reading as a sleep aid before he pulls the eye mask down over his eyes and inserts his ear plugs. My protocol was to keep talking until my eyes became weary, and suddenly I was gone. The best I could muster most nights on the *Explorer* was 'good night' or 'thanks'. I could see Marcus flip the page on the book he was reading out of the corner of my eye as I drifted off.

As kids growing up in Ireland, I never imagined this fierce competitor from a neighbouring county would one day take care of me in this manner. I am particularly proud that we didn't allow racing to dull our friendship. It could easily have turned out differently. We are the same age and have raced each other since we were fifteen. We went to rival US colleges; we ran the same event, but somehow, we managed to leave it on the track. Now thirty years later, here we were stepping in the shoes of Shackleton, Crean and McCarthy, albeit with one of us highly dependent on the other.

We spent the next couple of days exploring islands off the coast of the Antarctic. We visited penguins up close in their rookeries, and we saw monstrous elephant seals on beaches. One evening we encountered over a hundred whales feeding in a bay in multiple pods, all of these experiences against jaw-dropping gorgeous backdrops. The scenery is beyond spectacular and the scale unimaginable. As much as I enjoyed each of these adventures, I was distracted by the upcoming climbs.

First was Port Charcot on Booth Island. Port Charcot is the cove that the French explorer, Jean Baptiste Charcot, anchored in and set up his research station in 1910. He had a small cairn built on the highest point on the west end upon which flew the tricolour. The *Explorer* anchored a short distance off land, and we took the Zodiacs to shore. The sun was bright and the skies clear, allowing us to capture the majestic snow-covered mountains rising up from the ocean that was heavily spotted with broken bits of sea ice or pancake ice. The closer we got to shore, the more the shadow of the cairn towered over us. Close up, it was quite a climb.

We struggled up the embankment in our totally unsuitable boots. It had been very cold the previous night. The top layer of snow had hardened, shielding the softer snow underneath. The hard layer was thin like the veneer on a cheap dining room table and quickly yielded to our heavy Wellington boots. Suddenly, our feet were through the veneer, and we were knee deep in snow. Extracting our feet from the snow was no easy task, especially when the other foot was also on suspect ground. The guides had earlier forged a path and had tamped down the snow under their feet. The instructions were simple, stay on the path they had worn, and match their footprints. Marcus wisely recommended that we delay our departure to allow most of the others to complete the ascent first. This would allow maximum traffic, which would provide more compaction and render the trail more navigable.

Nonetheless, the trail was narrow; and although it had been trod on by the previous trekkers, I felt like a frog picking its way from lily pad to lily pad. I was more like a drunk frog with a hip displacement. The two walking sticks I brought were sadly ineffective, they kept burying into the snow. One in three stabs at the ground resulted in almost total submersion in the snow. Then I had to stop and yank the pole free.

There were distinct footprints and trying to match steps was tricky. I fell often, but the landings were soft and harmless as long as I fell uphill.

Thankfully, the guides had run the trail diagonally across the steepest tracks which made the climbs more manageable, but consequently longer. The trade-off made sense to me, but the round trip turned out to be approximately five kilometres.

We made it to the top and enjoyed the most stunning views of the entire trip. We lingered for quite a while and took some breathtaking pictures. I was exhilarated. It was like walking on hot coals; it may look ugly, but it is still quite a feat. Anyone watching would have discounted the achievement, but not me. I knew what I had been through. Now, I had climbed high in the Antarctic. I thought of the Irish explorers who had endured so much more. My accomplishment was minor in comparison, but to Marcus and me it was rewarding. Marcus gave me a hearty hug as we took pictures of the moment.

We couldn't savour it long. There was the not-small matter of getting back down. I was greatly concerned about the descent. I don't have tremendous control, and the decline demanded strong quad muscles. Each downward step required a braking action to combat gravity. If gravity was allowed to do its thing, I would hurtle down the hillside.

Also, I had to consider the optimum timing. If I waited too long, my medicine would be at its lowest ebb; I could experience freezing, a fitting name in this environment.

I turned to Marcus and said, 'I'm ready to go.'

He replied, 'We should rest longer, and let the others smooth out the trail some more.'

'I have to go now.'

'Relax, the boat is going nowhere.'

'But my medicine could run out. It generally wears out more quickly after a big exertion.'

'We brought back-up meds, right?'

'I did, but that takes a while to kick in.'

Marcus had seen enough nighttime freezing episodes, so he quickly concurred to a prompt departure. 'Let's go then.'

The plan was for Marcus to lead and act like a traffic-calming device. The first few hundred metres down the slope were the most precipitous. We moved very cautiously. I thought, 'What the hell am I doing up here?' Moreover, I was sporting rubber boots which were provided by the tour operator. They were far too slick and more suited to slushing around in the mud on a farm. The conditions under foot on Booth Island required crampons to safely navigate.

Marcus was fastidious in his role. He took very deliberate steps, making sure to firmly stamp on the ground and compact the snow as much as he could. I followed and oozed fearfulness as I painstakingly replicated each of his steps. I tried to keep my centre of gravity over my heels to prevent me from falling into Marcus and both of us from barrelling down the hillside. My quads were burning as we progressed. We rarely looked up to search for home. We stayed focused on each step, one at a time. Luckily, I have tons of experience living in the moment.

We eventually made it down, but there was still some flat ground to cover. Marcus, believing the job was done, slowed to take photographs of chinstrap penguins in a nearby rookery. I brushed past him, eager to complete the task while I still had adequate levels of Sinemet in my system. I pushed on across the remaining ground and arrived above the makeshift landing just as a Zodiac was pulling up. I was so keen to be done with the arduous test and fearful that the effort spent would draw out the Parkinson's symptoms that I immediately boarded the waiting Zodiac. Marcus, who was in hot pursuit, arrived at the Zodiac to find me sitting on the edge about to embark. He grabbed my hiking sticks and helped me aboard.

He naturally wondered why I was in such a big hurry. I tried to explain the obsessive nature of Parkinson's. You sometimes can see nothing but the task in front of you. No matter how dispensable the current task, you have to see it through. It is strange how strong a grip Parkinson's can have over your mind. It is not merely a movement disorder. Marcus was happy for me, but a little peeved that I hadn't heeded his advice to take more breaks and be more deliberate.

The next few days were spent with zodiac tours, kayaking adventures and endless encounters with chinstrap, gentoo and Adèlie penguins. We visited a former research station which appeared to be in pristine condition, or at least in the same condition as the day it was abandoned. That night was the hundredth anniversary of Ernest Shackleton's death, and one of the naturalists gave a wonderful presentation on the Irishman. He even had some original audio of the great man.

The ship sailed through the Lemaire Channel, which was covered in pack ice. The weather had warmed up enough to break up the sea ice to smaller flat pieces. This is referred to as pancake ice, unlike icebergs which are fuller and odd shaped and are land ice. We listened to the grinding noise and watched the hull cutting through the ice sheets as we cruised nonchalantly through the narrow passageway.

The next hike had added importance. It would mark the furthest south and the deepest within the Antarctic Peninsula we would adventure. It was a relatively short hike in distance, perhaps two kilometres long. It's difficult to gauge vertical distance. From the start, it was as steep as a black ski slope in Colorado. The guides again laid out a path, stomping their feet in the snow. There was no real skill involved in that work; it merely required an industrial touch. We watched them labour at the task from the ship and noted that the path was never vertical, rather it traversed the slope at a nearly horizontal angle with sixteen switchback turns. Each switchback created a severe change in direction.

The expedition leader advised that the conditions were similar to the previous hike, deep snow with a crusty cover. This time there was a twist; the crispy layer was slick as polished silver. On with the rubber boots, out with the hiking poles, and into the zodiac for the trip to land. The sun was bright and with hardly a cloud to be found in the sky, sunglasses were an absolute necessity. We even gambled on not taking our parkas; we knew we would be working hard to summit and would generate an excess of body heat.

Marcus was first off, and he tested the ice. His report was not encouraging. Upon further inspection, it turned out to be quite treacherous, especially in rubber boots. The guides had shovelled out a landing area and had cut steps into the bank of snow to access the surface we would be hiking on. They had laid towels on each step to offer traction against the Teflon-like surface. At the top of the artificial stairs, there was a bin to store our life jackets. We did not need extra weight to burden us on the climb. The first few steps were daunting and immediately required my fullest concentration. Marcus was concerned too and issued the same edict.

'Let's take our time, and for crying out loud follow in my footsteps.'

'I got it.'

I fell a couple of times on the first section. To which Marcus advised, 'Keep falling uphill, and we'll be fine.'

No matter how much I tried, it was almost impossible to extract my feet from the deep compacted snow. My boots would penetrate about eighteen inches searching for grip. Applying pressure to move my free foot, the

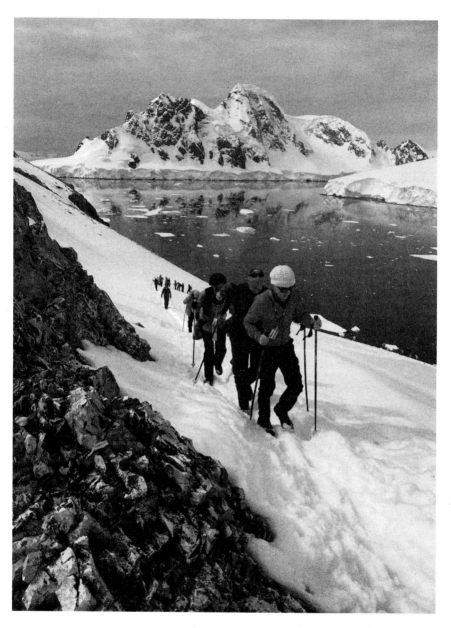

5 January 2022. Leading Marcus up a steep, icy incline on the Antarctic.

anchor foot would merely sink deeper. A number of times, Marcus had to drag me by my collar out of the snow.

He'd always counsel, 'You have to follow the footsteps.'

'I'm trying my best,' was the only response I could make.

Frequently, he would declare, 'Let's pull off the track at this corner and let these people by.'

We soldiered on, labouring over every step. There was a false summit, which was immensely disappointing. My quads were burning. I recalled vividly how I struggled coming down Port Charcot, and I remembered a quote I read about climbing. 'Getting to the top is optional, getting down is mandatory.' Don't get me wrong, this was no mountain, but to me it was a real beast. I thought, wouldn't it be wise to turn around? What if I can't get down? It was a mighty long way down, even from here. The last few turns Marcus went behind me. He feared that my legs were so tired I might fall over on the downhill side. On the last incline, I closed my eyes and just willed myself to the top.

My legs were shattered, and I lay down on the snow to restore my energy supplies. This climb was much steeper than Port Charcot, and I was genuinely frightened about the descent. I knew my legs were in real danger of quitting, so I agreed with Marcus to rest some more when he suggested it.

'Why don't we stay here a little longer and take a few pictures of the view? We can even get the ship in the background.'

I'm a sucker for a good picture so I agreed to stall our departure. 'Good idea, but we can't delay too long.'

'You need to be well rested. Getting down is going to be an effort.'

'Don't I know.'

'Wouldn't it make more sense to let the others go down first? They would firm up the trail more.'

We waited a little while before making our way to the edge. We were like skiers surveying a run before dropping in. Marcus reminded me. 'Okay, let's go; but I'm going first, and you're going to follow exactly in each of my footsteps.'

'Got it.'

'And one step at a time too.'

We began with a first awkward step and paused as Marcus levelled his footprint for my next step. We proceeded in this methodical fashion. By halfway down, my legs were screaming. It was constant braking with my quads that caused the fatigue. We noticed the traffic jam behind us, so we pulled over to let the others go around. We looked like an old lady holding up traffic in her Mini Cooper.

I took the opportunity to lie down on the snow. Strangely, so did a few others. Apparently, the icy conditions were a challenge for most, and they were happy with Marcus in the vanguard. We sat a while longer and took in the splendour of the Antarctic before setting off again, Marcus once more doing yeoman's work upfront or down below, depending on your perspective. Finally, we were down, and the crew had hot chocolate waiting for us.

We made some new friends on the voyage, one of whom had some real adventures to her credit; Kathy Sullivan has walked in space and been to the deepest part of the ocean. She could have easily discounted my little accomplishment, but she understood its significance to me. Wouldn't you know, that her family were Sullivans from Kenmare, just like mine. With our new company, we enjoyed another night on the seventh continent before heading back to the dreaded Drake Passage for our return to Ushuaia where we would make landfall on 9 January, exactly three years since my surgery and thirteen years since my first symptom.

## CHAPTER 19

# RESET EXPECTATIONS REGULARLY

That epic Antarctic adventure confirmed that many of the techniques I had been using to manage my Parkinson's worked. There was a clear link between achievement and wellbeing. The pride I felt at making it up those mountains was immeasurable. I know that my self-worth is closely aligned with my accomplishments, and I need to set manageable goals. In this case, the difficulty of getting down after the summit was a great reminder to choose my goals wisely. To ensure that I bend, but don't break.

The Antarctic also confirmed the necessity of discipline. In a strange way, the experience reminded me of boarding school. There was a rigorous schedule on board the ship that applied to all. We disembarked at the same time; we ate at the same time. There were strict protocols of how everything should be done, how to perform a wet landing and a dry landing with a Zodiac, when and where to wear a life vest. Rules and regulations are vital to the integrity of a group.

The most substantial revelation was the importance of incrementalisation. The only way I was getting down those mountains was by executing a one step at a time approach. It was paramount to place my boot precisely in Marcus's footprint. It was of the utmost importance to not look at the target, but to stay focused on the current step.

Parkinson's is like a glacier, slow moving but relentless. It keeps on coming regardless of what combat weapons you have at your disposal. As it moves, it calves massive chunks of ice. These icebergs are guerrilla fighters who spread out and attack secondary targets like the muscles involved in swallowing, blinking your eyes or shaping your mouth to speak clearly. Meanwhile, the glacier continues the central attack, eroding primary functions, stiffening your limbs, thwarting your movement, causing a tremor. It targets and attacks every imaginable function.

My biggest irritation with Parkinson's is it ruined my ability to parent. The distraction of daily Off Periods limited my capacity to be helpful to my kids. When I ought to have been there for them, I was in my foxhole fighting to survive. My brain was foggy and unable to process. Despite all the distractions, we raised three wonderful young men. To be accurate, Patty raised them. I largely spectated for the two youngest, especially Harry, who was only eleven when I got Parkinson's. He missed out on whatever fathering skills I possessed.

My sisters were just eleven when our father died, the same age as Harry on my diagnosis. My sisters barely remember their father, and I wonder what Harry's memories of me will be? Will he recall that I loved to read, to exercise or had a sense of humour?

Jack, and likely Colin too, will remember an occasion when their father's antics created a memorable moment. It was summertime and we were all in Limerick for a couple of weeks. Jack had made his First Communion earlier that spring, but at that Sunday's mass he would receive the Eucharist for the first time in Ireland. There is a peculiar habit in Ireland of church pews filling from the back forward. As a consequence, the front five or six rows can be empty. This was precisely the setup when we arrived at Christ the King parish church for 9am mass. The five of us entered and the only seats available were in the front rows. Jack chose the very front row in the middle aisle to sit. We stuck out like sore thumbs, kneeling there like an island in an ocean of empty seats. Word spread to the sacristy where the parish priest was preparing for the service. He immediately came out to see for himself.

Patty, seeing the priest approach in his white cassock, whispered, 'What have we gotten ourselves into now?'

The priest introduced himself. 'Hello. I'm Father Ryan. I'm the parish priest.'

'Hi, Father. I'm Frank O'Mara and this is my family.'

'Are you from the parish?'

'I am, my mother is sitting back there in the congregation.' Then I exclaimed the fateful words, 'Jack is making his First Communion in Ireland this morning.'

This seemed to throw Father Ryan off, but he regrouped and remarked, 'Well, we will have to make it special for him, won't we?'

We were already exposed, and that exposure was about to be amplified. I could feel my mother a few rows behind in seeming anonymity wondering what unwanted attention I had just drawn to the family.

When Father Ryan began Mass, he introduced us and remarked that this was Jack's First Communion and how nice it was that he had chosen Ireland and his grandmother's parish. He mentioned Jack in many prayers and included him in his homily. He spoke of First Holy Communion and its importance to a young man's spiritual journey. When it was time for the Eucharist, he instructed the congregation to remain seated while Jack and his family received the host. We were exhausted from embarrassment by the time Father Ryan dismissed us.

The highlight was yet to come. Congregants surrounded us in the vestibule. My mother, baffled at what she had just witnessed, reluctantly joined the throng offering their congratulations. Then a lady from her prayer group uttered these words, 'Mary, isn't it a terrible shame your grandson couldn't have dressed up for his First Holy Communion?'

Jack was not wearing a tie, but who would have imagined that one harmless remark from me could generate such controversy?

Of course, Jack and Colin have seen a firmer side too. The side that can't understand why you struggle with math or insists that you play a team sport. Harry has seen neither, at least none that he will remember. They each rely on their mother for counsel and guidance. Thanks to Patty, none of the three were truly short-changed. They are bright and caring and don't seem bothered by my measly parenting contribution. When I am with them there is always a willing arm for balance, a gentle tug if frozen or a voice to interpret my mumbling.

After years of fighting an endless war against the advancing foe, I am now much more guarded in my optimism. Unbridled positivity prevented me from accepting my fate and getting on with it. Parkinson's is my mortal enemy. It will always be, but my focus should be on learning to live with the condition rather than trying to outwit it. If I could just come to terms with my incapacities, I could suck the remaining sap from my tree of life. I have to stop thinking that I'll enjoy life again when I get over this ailment. I have changed irreversibly, but that doesn't mean I have been broken.

I need to dispense with defiance, or at least enough to let acceptance grow, but not so much that despondency gets a hold. I must moderate my acceptance levels annually to accommodate the disease progression and the

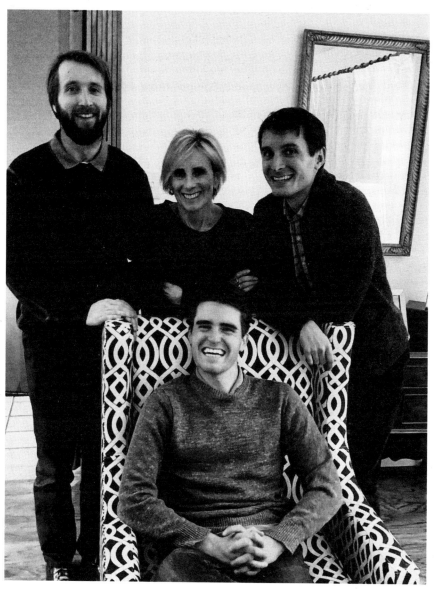

December 24, 2021 – Patty and our three boys. Clockwise from seated, Colin, Harry and Jack.

attendant incapacity. There's less disappointment that way. It's similar to trying to 'run your age' for a ten-kilometre race. Each year your target time slows by a minute. That seems reasonable.

Deep brain stimulation has returned much of my former self. Overall, I can honestly say my condition has improved, but am I better? It comes down to what is considered 'better'. Recently, I spoke with a friend, Bob Kennedy, and described my improvement to him. He was naturally delighted for me. At the end of the call, he said, 'I'm so glad you're better.' Then he corrected himself and said, 'Well, not *better*, I know you're never going to be better.' He continued, 'What do you say to someone with Parkinson's?'

'I know what you mean. "Better" works for me.'

It's true I'm never going to be 'better' in the sense that we use the term every day. But am I better? It all depends on your perspective. I'm never going to run again or ride my mountain bike or ski. However, I no longer have to deal with deadly neck cramps or dyskinesia and my overall condition has greatly improved.

Of course, I still encounter reminders that the future is uncertain. Just last night I struggled to get dressed and stared at the bed, frozen in place until Patty prodded me back to activity mode. If my future is dominated by those kinds of bothersome experiences, we will deal with them when we get there. We will not concern ourselves prematurely.

Meanwhile, there is a life to treasure and moments to relish. I am grateful for a wonderful and selfless wife and three loving sons. I am grateful for great siblings and friends and to anyone who has played a part in this twisted journey. I am grateful for this second chance. I am grateful to be better.

For too long, I avoided social contact because I feared my condition would alarm people or draw unwanted pity. But in the future, I will not worry about what others think of my tremor, or compromised walk or drooling or unintelligible speech, none of that matters one bit. I will park in a disabled dedicated spot without wondering who is watching.

I wish when I was younger somebody would have shared this bit of advice attributed to Will Rogers:

*When you are twenty, you care what everyone thinks,*

*When you are forty, you stop caring what everyone thinks, and*

*When you are sixty, you realise nobody was thinking about you*

*in the first place.*

How is my fate different than others, really? Some of us cruise to the finish line, while others struggle to make the distance. For those of us who struggle, better is possible, but better relative to what? Make sure you reach in that comparison. If you reach you grow, if you settle you decline.

I don't know what the future holds for me, but I am focused on what matters: living in the now, loving my family and friends. I will plan for the future, but I will never dwell on the future. I will never play a part I haven't been assigned. I will run the race one lap at a time, and I will not worry about the result. I will bend, but I will not break.

# DON'T FOOL YOURSELF

A couple of years after we sold AWCC to AT&T, I had dinner with Michael Prior, who was in town from Boston. I had not seen him in over a year. At that juncture, there were periods of every day when I still believed my symptoms weren't evident. I timed the dinner perfectly, right in the sweet spot of an On Period. The gods, however, were conspiring against me that evening. Or perhaps it was my loathing of one of my least favourite chores – putting gas in the car – that derailed my plans. I was driving to the restaurant when suddenly the car began shuddering; the tank was empty and I had to pull over on the shoulder. I couldn't rustle up a ride. Instead, I was forced to trudge to a gas station about six hundred metres away.

It was hot and I was already clammy from sitting in the car frantically calling different numbers for help. I called Michael and delayed our meal. I made my way to the gas station and bought a cheap plastic five-gallon can. I only filled it halfway because the weight and awkwardness made it difficult to carry. I began the trek back to the car. To my great relief I saw Patty driving toward me. She had picked up my voicemail and rushed to the scene of my silly blunder.

The whole ordeal took longer than I expected. I was sweaty, I was flustered, and I was late. The aggravation had exacerbated the symptoms and

I no longer had confidence that I could disguise them. I thought about cancelling, but I enjoyed Michael's company too much to do so. I reasoned that we were no longer business partners and if he saw through the façade what would it matter?

I had calmed down some by the time we sat down. We spoke about the massive effort it took to convert from the Verizon systems to brand new systems and how fortunate we were to win the hiring case. We discussed some of the individual key contributors including Lewis Langston, Brian Taylor, Scott Moody, Wade McGill and Lesa Handly, all of whom covered for me during my periods of incapacity.

My restlessness was still a distraction and I decided it was high time to explain myself. I broached the topic gingerly. 'There is something I should confess.'

Michael stopped me and said, 'You don't have to tell me. I already know.'

'What exactly do you know?' I responded.

'I knew you had Parkinson's.'

'You knew?'

'I can't say I was sure, but I was fairly certain.'

I had been flabbergasted by Michael Prior once before when he called me on the remote island of his ancestors to recruit me for the role at AWCC. Now for the second time, he floored me. The very thing I had tried so hard to hide was in plain view the whole time.

Then he added, 'My grandfather had Parkinson's, so I recognised the symptoms.'

'Why didn't you say?'

'Believe me, I would have, but you seemed to have everything under control.'

It turns out the only one I was fooling was myself. I had underestimated people's capacity to care. Many likely knew I was suffering. Perhaps they, like Michael, had some familiarity with the disease. Many probably suspected something was awry, but couldn't identify the condition. I misunderstood lack of 'reaching out' for lack of empathy.

I also underestimated people's capacity to trust me and value my opinion. Michael Prior knew and trusted me. Many at AWCC knew, but held me in similar regard. You can count my siblings, family and good friends in that. I am blessed to have so many people like them in my life. I didn't understand the true value of community and goodwill, that I had surrounded myself with enthusiastic and supportive people who insulate me from the worst and give me hope.

Thank you, you all are the reasons I bend, but don't break.

# ACKNOWLEDGEMENTS

The best guidance I received in writing this book was gleaned from Stephen King's *On Writing*. King cautions writers to walk away from the draft for a while, and let time provide fresh eyes and perspective. I did not. I imagine I couldn't because Parkinson's is a constant in my life now, and I can't seem to shake off the daily reminders. I was always updating the text with new revelations. In short, I was consumed by the disease and by writing about it. Consequently, there were innumerable drafts of this book. I'd like to thank some good friends who suffered through these early drafts: Scott Moody, John Hickman, Ian Bolger, Pierce O'Callaghan and Dave Taylor, thank you for seeing through misspellings and awkward transitions and nonetheless offering encouragement. To Steve Ovett, thank you for the most supportive note I have ever received on any topic. To others who read versions not ready for prime time, thank you.

A special thanks to my friend, Tom Vannah, who encouraged me to memorialise my journey. Tom helped me to find my voice, held me accountable on our Saturday morning calls and provided great composition suggestions.

Two articles in Irish newspapers, one by Sonia O'Sullivan in *The Irish Times*, the other by Cathal Dennehy in the *Irish Independent*, persuaded me that my story had relevance. I sent Sonia a copy and, to my surprise, she had read much of the book within short order. She contacted Helen Carr at O'Brien Press with whom she had previously collaborated. Helen read the three chapters I had already submitted and asked for the remainder.

Helen became my editor, my advocate and supporter. She provided direction, encouragement and made insightful suggestions.

Thanks to everyone at The O'Brien Press who supported this book in every capacity, especially Emma Byrne, for her design, Ruth Heneghan and Chloe Coome for their work on publicity, and Natasha Mac a'Bháird for proofreading.

I am deeply appreciative to a number of people not mentioned in the book from whom I learned so much: Kevin Beebe, Jeff Fox, Howard Hawes, Harry Bruns, John Ebner, John Koch and Dan Lohr from my Alltel days, Ger MacNamee, Frank Duhig, Declan O'Donoghue, coaches and mentors at St Munchin's College, John O'Donnell, Willie Logan and Ronnie Long at Limerick Athletic Club and Brian Taylor and Lesa Handly at AWCC. All of these individuals have one thing in common: they are givers and not takers.

Thanks also to my colleague Holly Larkin who read carefully and scrutinised for errors.

To Marcus for being a steadfast friend, confidant and fellow explorer.

I am forever grateful to Patty, my wife of thirty-four years who is not only a great companion, but also a punctuation ninja. Fortunately, she also has a good feel for composition and played a vital role in the construction of the book.

To my kids, I wish I could be a bigger presence in your lives. Keep on being who you are. I am proud of you.

# FRANK O'MARA: ATHLETIC ACHIEVEMENTS

Olympian: Los Angeles 1984 (1,500m), Seoul 1988 (5,000m), Barcelona 1992 (5,000m)

World Indoor Champion: Indianapolis 1987 (3,000m), Seville 1991 (3,000m)

NCAA (US Collegiate) Champion: Houston 1983 (1,500m)

USA Indoor Champion: Madison Square Garden 1989 (Mile)

Irish Champion: 1983, 1986, 1988, 1991 (1,500m), 1995 (5,000m)

World Record holder: 1985 4 x 1 Mile 15:49.08 (Coghlan, O'Sullivan, O'Mara, Flynn)

European Championship finalist: Stuttgart 1986 (1,500m), Helsinki 1994 (5,000m)

World Championship finalist: Rome, 1987

European Indoor Championships: Athens, 1985 (3,000m) 4th

Fifth Avenue Mile winner, 1985

**Personal Best Times:**

| | |
|---|---|
| 800m | 1:47.73 |
| 3,000m | 7:40.41 |
| 1,500m | 3:34.02 |

| | |
|---|---|
| 1 mile | 3:51.06 |
| 5,000m | 13:13.02 |
| 10,000m | 27.58.58 |

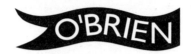
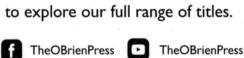